MCI and Alzheimer's Dementia

Clinical Essentials for Assessment and Treatment of Cognitive-Communication Disorders

MCI and Alzheimer's Dementia

Clinical Essentials for Assessment and Treatment of Cognitive-Communication Disorders

Kathryn A. Bayles, PhD, CCC-SLP

Cheryl K. Tomoeda, MS, CCC-SLP

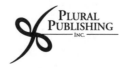

PLURAL
PUBLISHING
INC.

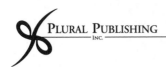
PLURAL PUBLISHING
INC.

5521 Ruffin Road
San Diego, CA 92123

e-mail: info@pluralpublishing.com
Web site: http://www.pluralpublishing.com

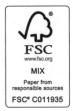

FSC
www.fsc.org
MIX
Paper from
responsible sources
FSC® C011935

Typeset in 10 ½ / 12 Palatino Book by Achorn International
Printed in the United States of America by McNaughton & Gunn, Inc.

Library of Congress Cataloging-in-Publication Data

Bayles, Kathryn A., 1942–
 MCI and Alzheimer's dementia: clinical essentials for
assessment and treatment of cognitive-communication disorders /
Kathryn Bayles, author, Cheryl Tomoeda, author.
       p. ; cm.
 Includes bibliographical references and index.
 ISBN-13: 978-1-59756-518-9 (alk. paper)
 ISBN-10: 1-59756-518-0 (alk. paper)
 I. Tomoeda, Cheryl K. II. Title.
 [DNLM: 1. Mild Cognitive Impairment—diagnosis. 2. Aged.
3. Alzheimer Disease—diagnosis. 4. Alzheimer Disease—therapy.
5. Mild Cognitive Impairment—therapy. WT 150]
 RC523
 616.8'31—dc23
                                        2013014051

Contents

Preface

This "mini-text," as we call it, is meant to provide students in training and practicing professionals the essential information needed to serve clients with minimal cognitive impairment (MCI) or clinically apparent Alzheimer's dementia (AD). Few communication sciences and disorders training programs have the luxury of fielding a course devoted entirely to the cognitive-communication disorders of dementia because of an already full master's curriculum. Nonetheless, students need an understanding of dementia to serve the profession's 2 fastest growing clinical populations. A chapter is insufficient to describe the syndromes of MCI and AD, their assessment and evidence-based treatment. A full-blown text is too much. This mini-text was developed to meet the needs of students and professors in a time-efficient and economical way. The focus is on Alzheimer's, the most common of the dementia-producing diseases, and its preclinical state, MCI.

The book comprises a meaty introduction, which gives readers an overview of cognition and memory, and 7 segments that cover the topics of MCI and AD, along with their assessment, a rationale for intervention, cognitive stimulation programming for MCI, direct interventions, and indirect interventions for AD. A summary of key points follows each segment.

Features of the mini-text that are timely are a chapter for speech-language pathologists on MCI, a population the profession is just recognizing, and a chapter by guest author Dr. Kimberly C. McCullough of the University of Central Arkansas, on cognitive intervention and MCI. Dr. McCullough is an award-winning teacher and expert on cognitive stimulation.

Introduction

Individuals with Alzheimer's disease (AD) are our fastest-growing clinical population, nationally and globally. In fact, every 4 seconds someone is diagnosed.[1,2] It was estimated in 2010 that 35.6 million individuals worldwide were affected. However, by the year 2030, 65.7 million people will have AD or a form of dementia, and 115.4 million will be affected by 2050.[3]

AD begins decades before it is clinically obvious, and once diagnosed it typically endures for many more years. Because the dementia syndrome is an inherent component of AD, its victims increasingly depend on others for survival. Most are cared for at home by family, typically with serious financial, social, and emotional consequences to all involved. Those patients and families who have the support of professionals have a higher quality of life.[4,5] Speech-language pathologists (SLPs) are among the professionals who can provide support to affected individuals and their families. As experts in language and communication science and the evaluation and treatment of communication disorders, SLPs are uniquely qualified to diagnose and treat the cognitive-communication disorders associated with the disease.

The goal of this book is to provide the clinically essential knowledge needed by SLPs and students in training to evaluate and treat individuals in the various stages of AD and counsel professional and personal caregivers. Toward that end, the first order of business is to answer the question "Why do individuals with AD have a communication disorder?" However, to answer that question, we need to first define communication.

Communication Defined

Communication is the sharing of information by means of a symbol system. When words are used, we call it linguistic communication, and nonlinguistic when other symbol systems are used, such as mathematical notation. To communicate, either linguistically or nonlinguistically, an individual must have an idea to share and a symbol system through which to express the idea. For example, symphony conductors communicate their ideas about tempo and loudness to orchestra members by moving a baton in prescribed ways. Baseball coaches communicate plays by hand signals to players. These are examples of nonlinguistic communication, and although nonlinguistic communication can be impaired as a consequence of AD, the focus of the SLP is on impairment in linguistic communication. Nonetheless, both nonlinguistic and linguistic communications are impaired in AD because both are cognitive processes for sharing information.

Another distinction critical to characterizing the effects of AD on communicative function is the difference between "speech" and "language." For our purposes, the term "speech" refers to the motor production of sounds and the term "language" refers to the symbol system by which sound is paired with meaning for a particular purpose. As previously noted, "linguistic communication" is the cognitive process of intentionally sharing ideas through language and in AD *the ability to communicate is affected more than speech and language.*

"Meaningful" communication requires the production and comprehension of ideas. The act of speaking, in and of itself, does not constitute communication because that which is spoken may be structurally and semantically meaningless. Similarly, knowing the grammar of a language does not ensure the ability to communicate. Communication occurs only when words have been structured in such a way that the listener comprehends the speaker's idea.

Now the question of why communication is affected in AD can be answered. Communication is affected because the pathophysiologic processes of AD disrupt information generation and processing. Patients are said to have a "cognitive-communication" problem because progressive deterioration of cognition interferes with communication. The fact is the production and comprehension of language cannot be separated from cognition. Consider just the simple act of naming an object—for example, a turnip. First you must perceive the features of the turnip. They must be matched to those in long-term memory for recognition to occur. Thereafter, you must form an intention to say the object's name. The linguistic representations of objects are part of long-term lexical memory and must be retrieved and brought to consciousness. Perhaps you are uncertain about how a turnip looks and therefore are unsure whether you are perceiving a turnip, parsnip, or rutabaga. If so, you have to decide whether to indicate your uncertainty. To articulate uncertainty about the object's name or identity, a motor plan must be formed. Thus, the simple act of object naming requires perception, access to long-term memory, association, recognition, lexical retrieval, decision making, motor planning, and self-monitoring.

Persons with AD have difficulty *producing* linguistic information because they have trouble thinking, generating, and ordering ideas, in part because information-processing capabilities of declarative and working memory systems are compromised,[6,7] in part because of progressive degradation of knowledge.[8,9] They have difficulty *comprehending* language because of deficits in the cognitive processes of perception, recognition, attention, memory, and degradation of knowledge.[10]

By understanding the brain systems that process information, their neural architecture and the relation of communication to cognition, clinicians can reasonably predict the types of cognitive-communicative disorders associated with damage to different brain areas. A brief review of cognition and memory is in order.

References

1. Alzheimer's Association. 2012 Alzheimer's disease facts and figures. *Alzh Dement*. 2012;8:131–168.
2. Ferri CP, Prince M, Brayne C, Brodaty H, Fratiglioni L. Global prevalence of dementia: a Delphi consensus study. *Lancet*. 2005; 366:2112–2117.
3. Prince M, Bryce R, Albanese E, Wimo A, Ribeiro W, Ferri CP. The global prevalence of dementia: a systematic review and metaanalysis. *Alzh Dement*. 2013;9:63–75.
4. Mittelman MS, Roth DL, Coon DW, Haley WE. Sustained benefit of supportive intervention for depressive symptoms in Alzheimer's caregivers. *Am J Psychiatry*. 2004;161:850–856.
5. Gaugler JE, Roth DL, Haley WE, Mittelman MS. Can counseling and support reduce Alzheimer's caregivers' burden and depressive symptoms during the transition to institutionalization? Results from the NYU caregiver intervention study. *J Am Geriatr Soc*. 2008;56:421–428.
6. Rogers SL, Friedman RB. The underlying mechanisms of semantic memory loss in Alzheimer's disease and semantic dementia. *Neuropsychologia*. 2008;46:12–21.
7. Hornberger M, Bell B, Graham KS, Rogers TT. Are judgments of semantics relatedness systematically impaired in Alzheimer's disease? *Neuropsychologia*. 2009;47:3084–3094.
8. Laisney M, Gifford B, Eustache F. [Semantic memory in Alzheimer's disease: contribution of semantic priming.] [in French] *Psychol Neuropsychiatr Vieil*. 2004;2:107–115.

9. Laisney M, Giffard B, Belliard S, de la Sayette V, Desgranges B, Eustache F. When the zebra loses its stripes: semantic priming in early Alzheimer's disease and semantic dementia. *Cortex.* 2011;47:35–46.

10. MacDonald MC, Almor A, Henderson VW, Kempler D, Andersen ES. Assessing working memory and language comprehension in Alzheimer's disease. *Brain Lang.* 2001;78:17–42.

Acknowledgments

A book, even a small one, requires the skills of many people. We thank Plural editors for their help and Angie Singh for encouragement. For her willingness to contribute a chapter on cognitive stimulation, we are grateful to Dr. Kimberly C. McCullough. Lesley Skinner has been a careful and caring proofreader and overseen the assembling of the book. Thanks also to tolerant family, who sacrificed weekend adventures for our deadlines.

Alzheimer's has touched our personal lives, and understanding it has been a focus of our professional lives. We are grateful to all the inspiring individuals with MCI and Alzheimer's disease who participated in our research and graciously shared their stories. It is our hope that the information in this book may help clinicians help them.

Contributors

Kimberly C. McCullough, PhD, CCC-SLP
Associate Professor
University of Central Arkansas
Chapter 6

Unit 1

Cognition, Memory, and Communication

Cognition and Memory

Cognition is a general term that refers to our information processing systems and stored knowledge. Basically, the human brain is a pattern recognition system, and memories are stored patterns. The processes that enable us to perceive and interpret patterns enable us to modify our behavior to ensure survival as well achieve more modest objectives.

The "Company of Cognition"

A helpful analogy for conceptualizing cognition is to think of it as a large company whose mission is to analyze sensation, detect and remember regularities in incoming sensory information, and use experience to guide behavior. The "company of cognition" has numerous departments whose personnel perform unique functions but nonetheless work in parallel with personnel in other departments. Each department is responsible for analyzing a certain kind of sensory input (auditory, visual, tactile, gustatory, and olfactory). For example, there is a department for processing auditory sensations, one for processing visual stimuli, and so on. Ultimately, all departments report to an executive division that analyzes information, makes decisions, and plans action.

Each department in the "company of cognition" has unique neural architecture. The department that processes auditory sensations is the province of the temporal lobes. Processing visual sensations is the province of the occipital lobes, and somatic sensations are processed by the parietal lobes. The frontal lobes make decisions and carry out executive functions. All departments share information by virtue of fiber tracts connecting them, and all send their output via fiber tracts to the frontal lobes. In similar fashion, the lobes of the brain are connected to the limbic system, which is responsible for linking emotion with sensation. The limbic system, in turn, is linked to the frontal executive system.

Thinking of cognition as a company, with many departments working together to process information, is similar to how Alexander Luria,[1] the late renowned Soviet psychologist, described cognitive functioning. In Luria's 3-unit model, one neural unit governs arousal and tone, another unit processes sensory information, and a third makes decisions and initiates action. The integrity of all 3 units is essential to normal cognitive functioning. If the level of arousal is poor, then information processing by other units is compromised. If a sensory processing system is damaged, individuals can develop agnosias and/or other processing deficits. When the executive unit is dysfunctional, judgment, attention, and decision making are compromised.

Memory Defined

Memory is not a unitary phenomenon,[2-4] nor does it serve a single psychological function. Consider that you have memory for facts, faces, sensations, various procedures, music, symbol systems, words, and contexts. In fact, many memory systems exist.[2,5-9] A popular and clinically useful schema[10] for characterizing the types of memory is shown in Figure 1–1. These different memory systems rely on distinct neurologic substrates, process different kinds of information, and have different rules of operation. Of great importance to clinicians is that these systems can be separately impaired by neurologic disease and injury. Thus, clinicians need an understanding of the different memory systems, their operational principles, and neural architecture to understand why an individual with a particular type and distribution of neuropathology has certain symptomatology.

Sensory Memory

At the earliest stage of information processing is the registration of sensation. Sensations are received by our peripheral receptor

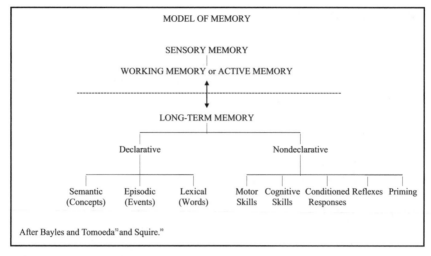

Figure 1–1. A model of memory.[10,52]

organs (eg, eyes, ears, chemical receptors) and interpreted in sensory cortices. A helpful way to think about sensory memory is as a playback system in which incoming sensory information is sustained long enough that it can be reviewed for further processing.[11] The auditory playback system is known as *echoic memory*. The visual playback system is called *iconic memory*.

Sensory Memory: A Preattentive System

The term *sensory memory* applies to sensations that occur at the level of the peripheral receptor organs before they are consciously realized.[12–14] Higher order attentional processes bring some sensations to consciousness, though not all. As you might suspect, information in sensory memory rapidly decays to make way for the representation of new incoming sensations. The duration of sensory memory is estimated to range from a third of 1 second to as long as 2 seconds.[15–16]

When an individual has a deficit in a peripheral receptor organ, sensation is altered and the quality of information coming from the environment is degraded. To facilitate sensory memory, clinicians must ensure that clients with sensory impairments, such as impaired vision or hearing, wear their glasses and hearing aids.

Working Memory

When sensations are consciously realized, they are in what is widely known as working memory. Alan Baddeley[17] introduced the term *working memory* to refer to both information in conscious awareness and the processes active in the conscious awake person. The term is popular because it implies that much work is going on in consciousness, and indeed there is. One activity is the focusing of attention that enables individuals to bring certain sensations to consciousness. But attention is only one of many processes referred to by the term *working memory*. Consider that when sensation is brought to consciousness, it must be interpreted. Multiple working memory subsystems enable us to review newly received information. Two subsystems that are of particular relevance to speech-language pathologists are the *articulatory/phonological loop* and the *visuospatial sketchpad*. The articulatory/phonological loop makes possible the subvocal rehearsal of that which we have just heard, and the visuospatial sketchpad enables us to recirculate, in our "mind's eye," that which we have just seen.

To interpret new information, we rely on previous experience. Thus, working memory must activate past experience and bring that knowledge to consciousness. Generally, decisions must be made about the new information the organism is receiving. Baddeley[17] called the decision-making component of working memory the *central executive*. The central executive system focuses attention, encodes information, retrieves information from long-term stores, plans action, and solves problems.

When information in working memory is encoded in long-term memory, it is linked with other, similar memories. For example, new concepts are linked with those previously learned, new procedures are linked with other procedures, and new words with other words. The 2-way arrows in Figure 1–1 signify that information is transferred from working memory to long-term memory and is retrieved from long-term memory when needed. Encoding and retrieval are carried out by the working memory system.

Active Memory

A synonym for working memory is active memory. It is whatever is on your mind. Said another way, it is what you are thinking about. Working memory can be conceptualized as containing buffers that store incoming sensory information, but the buffers have a limited capacity. In a classic experiment in 1956, Miller[18] demonstrated that the buffer span capacity of working memory is, on average, 7 ± 2 units of unrelated information. When the amount of information exceeds buffer capacity, some falls from consciousness. The terms used to refer to the buffer span capacity of an individual's working memory are *short-term memory, primary memory,* or *memory span.* Encoded information that has fallen from consciousness, regardless of whether it was a few seconds or years ago, is long-term memory.[19] Many people mistakenly refer to information that fell from consciousness a short time ago as short-term memory. However, short-term memory refers to only the amount of information that can be *held* in consciousness. Long-term memory refers to information that has fallen from consciousness even if it was a short time ago.

Neural Substrates of Working Memory

As you may have surmised, the frontal lobes are essential to working memory, particularly prefrontal regions which are extensively connected with the sensory processing systems of the brain and structures that underlie emotion. Eichenbaum[20] notes that the prefrontal cortex has the capacity to hold items in consciousness for manipulation and the encoding of stimuli and events. Its subdivisions are "highly connected with one another and with posterior areas of the cortex to operate as a complex and widespread network for conscious control over memory and other intellectual functions" (p. 336). The dorsolateral prefrontal cortex bilaterally is the "CEO" of the company of cognition.[21]

The articulatory/phonological loop is subserved by Broca's area and surrounding cortex as well as the inferior parietal and inferior temporal cortices. The visuospatial sketchpad is supported by the occipito/parietal cortex, which mediates the visual/spatial components, respectively.[22] Individuals with dementia typically have damage to the frontal lobes and structures that input to the frontal lobes. As a consequence, the functioning of working memory is compromised in dementia.

Long-Term Memory

Long-term memory is commonly dichotomized as *declarative* or *nondeclarative* knowledge.[10] Declarative knowledge is factual information that can be declared. A synonym for declarative memory is explicit memory because fact knowledge can be made explicit. Nondeclarative memory is a broader term referring to movement or motor memory, certain cognitive skills, priming, conditioned responses, and reflexes.

Declarative Memory

Declarative knowledge, or fact memory, can be subdivided into 3 related systems: semantic memory (SM), episodic memory (EM), and lexical memory (LM).

Semantic Memory.

Concept: Elemental Unit. SM is that domain in the nervous system in which conceptual knowledge is represented. The term semantic memory was introduced by Quillian,[23] who proposed a theory of information processing that included a long-term store of conceptual knowledge.[24-26] Concepts are constructs we form about the world based on our experiences. As Smith and Medin wrote in their book about categories and concepts,[27,p1] "Without concepts, mental life would be chaotic. If we perceived each entity as unique, we would be overwhelmed by the sheer diversity of what we experience and unable to remember more than a minute fraction of what we encounter."

The word "semantic" in the term *semantic memory* may make some readers think that the contents of SM are words. However, the elemental unit of SM is theorized to be the concept, not the word. If you find that hard to accept, consider that humans can conceptualize things for which they have no words. For example, you can conceptualize the following for which no word exists: "an amorphous mass of gelatinous material about the size of a basketball seeming to have a self-contained propulsion system that enables it to continually change shape."

Other evidence that the units of SM are not in one-to-one correspondence with words is that many concepts can be referred to by a single word—for example, "net." "Net" is associated with the concept of a tennis court barrier, a fisherman's tool, what is left after expenses, and a material used to make prom formals, just to name a few of its referents. Conversely, one concept can be associated with many words. For example, the concept of religion is associated with

Taoism, Protestantism, Catholicism, Judaism, Buddhism, Islam, and so forth.

Concepts can be activated by words, but conceptual activation can result from nonlinguistic stimuli as well—from objects and pictures, for example. A picture of a parallelogram may activate the spatial concepts of parallel lines and opposing lines of equal length but not the word "parallelogram." Every day, individuals obtain new information by nonlinguistic means, and unless the need arises, much of this knowledge is never given linguistic representation. Consider that individuals who are profoundly deaf develop concepts without forming a linguistic representation for them. When a deaf child touches a hot stove, the concept of hot is encoded; however, without language training, the child will never develop the word "hot." Also, consider that an individual can lose the word for a concept without losing the concept, as can an individual with anomic aphasia.

Words certainly help us conceptualize and indeed are so helpful that much thinking is done in words. However, when information is stored, the words that conveyed the information are generally forgotten; instead, we remember the concepts expressed by the words.

SM is a hierarchically organized network of associations such that related concepts are linked. Thus, when the concept of a storm is activated, the related concepts of wind, rain, and lightning are also activated. Although the concept is the elemental structural unit of SM, it is not the only unit. Propositions and schemata, which are combinations of concepts, also have representation.

Proposition. A *proposition* can be defined as a relational expression. It is grammatically analogous to a clause and contains a relational term, such as a verb, and one or more nouns or noun phrases that function as subjects and objects of the relation. For example, the following are propositions:

Children dress up in costumes on Halloween.

Global warming is affecting weather.

Broccoli is a nutritious vegetable.

These propositions have been given linguistic representation, though not all propositions are translated into words.

Considerable evidence exists for the psychological reality of propositions. For example, regardless of the grammatical form of a sentence, it is reducible to the same constituent propositions; that is, it makes no difference whether the propositions are couched in a complex syntactic frame, a compound construction, or a simple construction.[28,29] People can recognize when 2 sentences or clauses are equivalent paraphrases because they perceive the relational expression, or proposition, contained in them. The following 2 sentences, which are equivalent paraphrases, illustrate this fact:

1. He desires to purchase an acre of land with a panoramic view of Tucson.
2. He really wants to buy an acre-sized lot with a valley-wide view of the "Old Pueblo."

Sachs[30] demonstrated that people remember propositions (or conceptual meaning) and ultimately forget the grammatical form in which they were expressed. Some investigators have demonstrated that it is the number of propositions, rather than the number of words, that affects the memorability of the meaning of a sentence.[31,32]

Schemata. A *schema* is an attentional set formed by the simultaneous activation of a group of related concepts (Figure 1–2). Schemata are another structural unit of SM. People have schemata

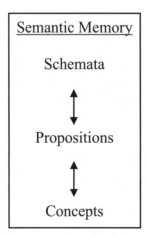

Figure 1–2. Semantic memory: a hierarchically organized representational system.

for a multitude of activities—for example, packing a carry-on bag for an airplane, being a member of a wedding party, using a cell phone, making an appointment with a doctor.

The process of building new schemata involves learning the associations between/among a particular set of concepts and propositions. For example, individuals exposed to the game of golf learn a host of propositions—for example, that certain clothes and shoes are worn when playing golf, that the angle of the club face influences the trajectory of the golf ball, that different clubs are used for different kinds of shots, that the person who had the fewest strokes on the previous hole hits first on the new hole, and that it is rude to talk when someone is hitting the ball. By playing golf, the schema is strengthened until the conventions of golf become second nature. Schemata help us know what to expect and guide our behavior.

Episodic Memory. *Episodic Memory* (EM) is the system that "receives and stores information about temporally dated episodes or events, and temporal-spatial relations among them."[33,p223] One way to think about episodic memory is that it is SM plus a context. An example may make this point clear. Consider that golf is a concept represented in SM. Now, let's assume that you played golf last Sunday morning. That was an event, an episode. If you can remember the event of having played golf last Sunday morning, that is EM. Notice that a context, "last Sunday morning," was added to the conceptual base of golf as a game in the EM example. SM is what you *know*: you know golf is a game; EM is an event you can *remember*: playing golf last Sunday. Likely you do not remember the context in which you learned that golf is a game—it is just something you know, like knowing that an apple is a fruit. But being able to remember the last time you played golf or ate an apple is EM.

A synonym for EM is chronologic memory. EM enables us to travel back in time to recall past events. It is more fragile than SM. In fact, we forget most of the events of our lives. Likely you cannot remember what you ate for dinner on the 25th of last month, or the color of the car parked next to yours in the parking lot last Friday, or how the napkins were arranged at the last dinner party you attended. Insignificant events are forgotten.

Lexical Memory. *Lexical Memory* (LM) is our knowledge of words, their form and meaning. Certainly concepts and their linguistic representations are intimately connected; however, people can have concepts for which they have no lexical representation, and lexical information can be impaired without impairment of conceptual knowledge. Individuals with aphasia typically have preserved conceptual knowledge but struggle with lexical representations. Word knowledge also includes knowledge of the rules for composing syntactically correct and grammatical sentences. These operations are theorized to rely on the neural systems that support procedural memory.

Neural Substrates of Declarative Memory

The declarative memory system is supported by 3 primary components: the cortex, the parahippocampal region, and the hippocampus. Together, these brain regions enable us to acquire factual knowledge and remember events. Recall that the cortex is the endpoint for incoming sensory information. Within each sensory modality (or lobe), sensations are analyzed by a hierarchy of cells that perform increasingly complex analyses. The results of the analyses are sent to association areas of the cortex that have the capacity to form multimodal representations of information. These multimodal association areas have extensive inputs to the medial temporal lobes and parahippocampal regions. The parahippocampal region is able to sustain this input for short periods of time, thereby enabling the hippocampus to "process comparisons among the various current stimuli and events and between current stimuli and representations of previous stimuli and events."[20,p235] It is the hippocampus that makes it possible to add new cortical representations of information or restructure existing cortical representations.[34] Cells in the hippocampi have the capacity for long-term potentiation, meaning they can stay active for extended periods of time, enabling them to replay information recently received. The replay of information during sleep provides the cortex the opportunity to repeatedly strengthen the link between new, recently experienced sensations and previously existing representations of knowledge. Because the hippocampi function like an index to link new, incoming information with previously learned information, individuals with hippocampal damage have difficulty remembering recent events and making new SM.

Just anterior to the hippocampi lie the amygdalae, which are important in the processing of emotion.[35–37] There is strong evidence that the amygdalae modulate declarative memory on the basis of emotion.[35,38] Emery[11] theorizes that autobiographical memory developed phylogenetically from emotional memory, a theory that has considerable appeal because the emotional significance of an event greatly influences its memorability. Emery's research, from a life themes study, indicates that episodic memory may be coded in both pictures (visual code) and words (verbal code).[11]

Factual knowledge is said to be "distributed" throughout the cortex. That is, it is not stored in a single area. Take, for example, your fact knowledge of your maternal grandmother. You have knowledge of what she looks like, how her voice sounds, what she smells like, how she feels when you hug her, as well as event knowledge about times you have spent with her. This diverse knowledge is not represented in one cell or cell assembly. Rather, it is believed that your knowledge of how grandmother looks has representation in visual association cortex and how her voice sounds in auditory association cortex and so on. Multimodal association cortex, where information from the various sensory processing systems converges, contains a more complex representation of grandmother. This explanation is very simplistic but makes the point that conceptual knowledge is distributed across cortical sensory association areas. For a more in-depth account of the brain system that supports declarative memory, the reader is referred to *The Cognitive Neuroscience of Memory* by Eichenbaum.[2]

Word knowledge is fact knowledge and as such is supported by the neural systems that underlie declarative memory.[39] Although lexical knowledge is represented in both cerebral hemispheres, the left temporal lobe is key in the processing of word forms and meaning in both expressive and receptive language tasks.[40–43] By studying the naming errors of people with brain damage and brain activation patterns of neurologically normal adults during picture naming, Damasio et al[44] identified 3 brain regions of particular importance to word knowledge: the anterior inferior temporal pole, the middle part of the inferior temporal gyrus, and the posterior region of the temporal lobe. However, not all lexical operations rely on the same temporal lobe structures. Phonological processing relies on the middle and posterior regions of the superior temporal cortex, whereas conceptual-semantic knowledge appears reliant on areas in front of and below these areas.[45,46] Other brain structures also support lexical processing, among them subcortical and cerebellar structures. Word knowledge also includes knowledge of the rules for composing syntactically correct and grammatical sentences. These operations are theorized to rely on the neural systems that support procedural memory. For an overview, see Ullman's 2007 chapter in the work edited by Gaskell.[47]

Nondeclarative Memory

As previously mentioned, *nondeclarative memory* is a general term referring to several kinds of memory and processes: motor skills, cognitive skills, priming, conditioned responses, and reflexes (non-associative learning). A characteristic of these different types of non-declarative memory is that they are strengthened by repetition and practice.

Motor Skill Memory. *Motor skill memory* refers to motor proce-dures that are learned and the processes that support them. Ex-amples of motor skill memory are riding a bicycle, driving a car, typing, and articulating (Figure 1–3). Unlike declarative memory, which comprises factual knowledge that can be stated, motor pro-cedural memory refers to the *performance* of an action. One can think about the mechanics of driving a car, but that is not procedural memory. Motor procedural memory is exhibited in the *act* of driv-ing the car. One has knowledge about how to ski or play tennis, but

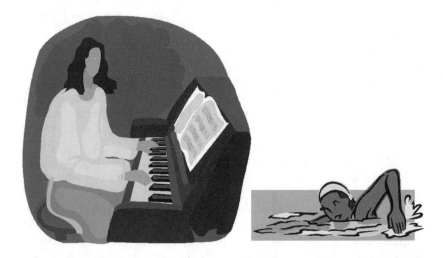

Figure 1–3A–B. Examples of motor skill memory include playing a piano and swimming.

motor procedural memory is evident only when one actually skis or hits the tennis ball.

    Neural Substrate of Motor Skill Memory. Motor skill memory (also known as motor procedural memory) is supported by the corticostriatal system, including premotor and motor cortex, basal ganglia, and cerebellum.[48–50]

Cognitive Skill Memory. *Cognitive skill memory* is an umbrella term for various cognitive procedures that occur without conscious awareness. Examples are mirror-reversed reading and recognizing holographic images nested in pictures. The neural substrates for various cognitive skills differ, making it impossible to specify a single neural architecture.

Priming. *Priming* is the facilitation of performance as a consequence of previous experience with a stimulus and is typically measured in terms of accuracy of judgment or latency of response. Priming can be conceptual or perceptual. Conceptual priming is the spreading of activation between or among related concepts. An example of conceptual priming is the activation of the concepts of cold, hard, and water when we hear the word "ice."

    In perceptual priming, the prior exposure to perceptual features of the stimulus facilitates the response. For example, the word "cake" may be activated by having previously seen the word "cake" or a word similar in appearance, such as "make."

    Neural Substrates of Priming. Priming occurs in the neocortex, but certain subcortical structures may facilitate priming, notably the basal ganglia. The areas of cortex involved depend on the nature of the stimulus, that is, whether it is a concept or a set of perceptual features. When the stimulus is visual, areas of the occipital lobe and/or inferior temporal lobe are involved. When the stimulus is auditory, both the left and right auditory cortices are involved. The left auditory cortex processes cues related to phonologic information; the right auditory cortex processes cues related to the speaker's voice.

Habits and Conditioned Behaviors. *Habits* are chains of behavioral events. The events in the chain are associated with each other such that the execution of one behavior triggers the next behavior.

Most of us have a chain of behaviors we follow upon awakening and before we go to bed. We can carry out this routine while thinking about something else. Humans can develop habits because of the brain's capacity to form associations between repeated events. In fact, Eichenbaum[2] defines habit as "an acquired and well-practiced response to a particular stimulus."

Conditioned behaviors are automatically produced in response to a particular stimulus or set of stimuli. The behavior is associated with the stimulus and reinforced by the events subsequent to the behavior or the eradication of an unpleasant antecedent event. An example is feeling afraid when approached by a growling dog.

Neural Substrates of Habit Memory and Conditioned Behaviors.

The corticostriatal system, in particular the striatum, underlies the formation of habits.[51] Eichenbaum[2] explains that the striatum receives cortical sensory input and has direct motor outputs that make possible the association of stimuli with behavioral outputs. The striatum also has pathways for reward signals that enhance the association of stimuli and responses. Individuals with damage to the striatum are impaired in developing stimulus-response sequences.

The cerebellum is important in motor conditioning.[10] Its circuitry enables it to make a topographic representation of the entire body surface because it receives vestibular, visual, and auditory inputs and has complex connections with the brainstem.[2] Individuals with damage to the cerebellum are impaired in the acquisition of classically conditioned responses.

Relation of Cognition and Memory to Communication

Production of Linguistic Information

Ideation begins the process of producing meaningful linguistic output. The ideas that people communicate can be reduced to concepts represented in their SM. Once an idea or idea sequence has been formulated, it must be translated into a symbol system for linguistic communication to occur. A point to be underscored is that a translation process occurs; that is, ideation and thinking may be done in a different language than is seen on the written page or heard in a lecture. The brain appears to have a language of its own, a machine language, or as Fodor[53] says, a language of thought, the output of which is translatable into human natural language. To utter or write an idea, we rely on complex motor skills (articulation or writing) that are forms of nondeclarative procedural memory. To ensure that what we say is what we intended to say, we monitor our utterances and make judgments about them. Thus, the production of linguistically expressed information uses SM, LM, working memory, motor procedural memory, and the central executive system. Although this is an oversimplification of what occurs in producing language, it makes the point that our *cognitive-memorial systems underlie communication*.

Comprehension of Linguistic Information

Linguistic comprehension ultimately involves deriving the right concepts and propositions. Said another way, it involves activation of the intended concepts in LM and SM. Like linguistic production, linguistic comprehension is the product of sequential and parallel processes involving many parts of the nervous system. For example, the perception of a spoken concept (word) or proposition (sentence) can be traced from its detection by the auditory system, in which feature, segmental, and word analyses occur, to the level of SM and consciousness. Through their nervous system journey, linguistic stimuli undergo lexical, structural, and logical analyses, the output of which is awareness of the intended concept or proposition. Additionally, the context in which a communicative exchange occurs influences the interpretation of information exchanged. "Context" refers to the physical setting, emotional climate, social organization between participants, and the purpose of the communicative exchange. Tracking these variables is a complex constructive process, and participants in a communicative exchange must attend to phonetic and paraverbal features such as pitch, intonation, gestures, and facial expressions, as well as the physical setting.

Now the question of why communication is affected in Alzheimer's disease can be answered. Communication is affected because the pathophysiologic processes of Alzheimer's disease disrupt information generation and processing. Patients are said to have a "cognitive-communication" problem because progressive deterioration of cognition interferes with communication. The fact is that the production and comprehension of language cannot be separated from cognition.

Summary of Important Points

- Communication is the sharing of information by means of a symbol system and is a manifestation of cognition.
- Persons with dementia have trouble with intentional communication because by definition they have multiple cognitive deficits.
- Cognition is stored knowledge and the processes for making and manipulating knowledge.
- Cognition can be likened to a large company whose mission is to analyze sensation, detect and remember regularities in incoming sensory information, and use experience to guide behavior.
- Memory can also be defined as stored knowledge and the processes for making and manipulating it.
- Humans have many memory systems, each with a distinct neural architecture that can be separately impaired by trauma or disease.
- Sensory memory is the brief registration of sensation at the level of the peripheral receptor organ. It is preattentive, and sensations rapidly fade, making way for new sensations.
- Working memory is information in conscious awareness and the processes active in the reception, encoding, and retrieving of information.
- Much work goes on in working memory that is directed by a central executive that enables us to make decisions and plan action.
- Long-term memory can be dichotomized as declarative knowledge and nondeclarative knowledge.
- Declarative memory is fact memory and can be subdivided into semantic, episodic, and lexical memory.
- Semantic memory comprises our conceptual knowledge; it is what we know. The elemental unit is the concept.
- Episodic memory enables us to remember the events of our life. It is our autobiographical memory and the most fragile of the memory systems.
- Lexical memory is our memory for words, their referents and meaning, spelling, and pronunciation.
- *Nondeclarative memory* is a general term that refers to several kinds of memory: skills (motor and cognitive), habits, priming, conditioned responses, and reflexes.
- Motor skill memory is often referred to as procedural memory. It is realized in the doing of a skill such as driving a car or hitting a tennis ball.

- Cognitive skill memory refers to myriad cognitive operations that occur without conscious awareness, one of which is mirror-reversed reading.
- Priming is the facilitation of performance as a consequence of previous experience with a stimulus or its associates. Priming can be conceptual or perceptual.
- Habits are chains of behavioral events in which the execution of one behavior triggers the next behavior.
- The production and comprehension of linguistic information cannot be separated from cognition but rather reflect cognition.
- Persons with dementia have difficulty producing linguistic information because they have trouble thinking, generating, and ordering ideas. They have difficulty comprehending language because of deficits in cognitive processes and degradation and loss of knowledge.
- With an understanding of the types of memory and their neural substrates, clinicians can reasonably predict the cognitive-communicative disorders associated with damage to different brain areas.

References

1. Luria A. *The Working Brain*. New York, NY: Basic Books; 1973.
2. Eichenbaum H. *The Cognitive Neuroscience of Memory*. 2nd ed. New York, NY: Oxford University Press; 2012.
3. Schacter DL, Wagner AD, Buckner RL. Memory systems of 1999. In: Tulving E, Craik FIM, eds, *Oxford Handbook of Memory*. New York, NY: Oxford University Press; 2000:627–643.
4. Squire LR, Stark CEL, Clark RE. The medial temporal lobe. *Ann Rev Neurosci*. 2004;27:279–306.
5. Cohen JN, Squire L. Preserved learning and retention of pattern-analyzing skill in amnesia: dissociation of "knowing how" and "knowing that." *Science*. 1980;210:207–209.
6. Gaffan D. Recognition impaired and association intact in the memory of monkeys after transection of the fornix. *J Comp Physiol Psych*. 1974;86:1100–1109.
7. Hirsh R. The hippocampus and contextual retrieval from memory: a theory. *Behav Biol*. 1974;12:421–444.
8. Nadel L, O'Keefe J. The hippocampus in pieces and patches: an essay on modes of explanation in physiological psychology. In: Bellairs R, Gray EG, eds, *Essays on the Nervous System. A Festschrift for JZ Young*. Oxford, UK: Clarendon Press; 1974.

9. Schacter DL. Multiple forms of memory in humans and animals. In: Weingerger N, McGaugh J, Lynch G, eds, *Memory Systems of the Brain: Animal and Human Cognitive Processes*. New York, NY: Guilford Press; 1985:351–379.

10. Squire LR. Memory systems of the brain: a brief history and current perspective. *Neurobiol Learn Mem*. 2004;82:171–177.

11. Emery VOB. "Retrophylogenesis" of memory in dementia of the Alzheimer type. In: Emery VOB, Oxman TE, eds, *Dementia: Presentation, Differential Diagnosis, and Nosology*. Baltimore, MD: John Hopkins University Press; 2003:177–236.

12. Downar J, Crawley AP, Mikulis DJ, Davis KD. A multimodal cortical network for the detection of changes in the sensory environment. *Nat Neurosci*. 2000;3:277–283.

13. Tanaka E, Kida T, Inui K, Kakiqi R. Change-driven cortical activation in multisensory environments: an MEG study. *Neuroimage*. 2009;24:464–474.

14. Tanaka E, Inui K, Kida T, Kakiqi R. Common cortical responses evoked by appearance, disappearance, and change of the human face. *BMC Neurosci*. 2009;10:38.

15. Dick AO. Iconic memory and its relation to perceptual processes and other memory mechanisms. *Percept Psychophys*. 1974; 16:575–596.

16. Harrell M, Parente F, Bellingrath EG, Lisicia KA. *Cognitive Rehabilitation of Memory: A Practical Guide*. Gaithersburg, MD: Aspen; 1992.

17. Baddeley AD. *Working Memory*. Oxford, UK: Clarendon Press; 1986.

18. Miller, AG. The magical number seven, plus or minus two: some limits on our capacity for processing information. *Psychological Review*,1956;63:81–97.

19. James W. *The Principles of Psychology*. New York, NY: H. Holt & Company; 1890.

20. Eichenbaum H. *The Cognitive Neuroscience of Memory*. Cambridge, UK: Oxford University Press; 2002.

21. Smith EE, Jonides J. Storage and executive processes in the frontal lobes. *Science*. 1999;283:1657–1661.

22. Baddeley AD. Working memory: looking back and looking forward. *Nat Rev Neurosci*. 2003;4:829–839.

23. Quillian MR. Semantic memory. Unpublished doctoral dissertation. Carnegie Institute of Technology; 1966. Reprinted in part in Minsky M, ed, *Semantic Information Processing*. Cambridge, MA: MIT Press; 1968.

24. Cohen G. *The Psychology of Cognition.* 2nd ed. New York, NY: Academic Press; 1983.
25. Tulving E. Episodic and semantic memory. In: Tulving E, Donaldson W, eds, *Organization of Memory.* New York, NY: Academic Press; 1972:381–403.
26. Wickelgren WA. *Cognitive Psychology.* Englewood Cliffs, NJ: Prentice-Hall; 1979.
27. Smith EE, Medin DL. *Categories and Concepts.* Cambridge, MA: Harvard University Press; 1981.
28. Franks JJ, Bransford JD. Memory for syntactic form as a function of semantic context. *J Exp Psych.* 1974;103:1037–1039.
29. Wang MD. Frequency effects in the abstraction of linguistic ideas. *Bull Psychonom Soc.* 1977;9:303–306.
30. Sachs JS. Recognition memory for syntactic and semantic aspects of connected discourse. *Percep Psychophys.* 1967;2:437–444.
31. Kintsch W, Glass G. Effects of propositional structure upon sentence recall. In: Kintsch W, ed, *The Representation of Meaning in Memory.* Hillsdale, NJ: Lawrence Erlbaum Associates; 1974:140–151.
32. Rochon E, Waters GS, Caplan D. Sentence comprehension in patients with Alzheimer's disease. *Brain Lang.* 1994;46:329–349.
33. Tulving E. Elements of episodic memory (precis). *Behav Brain Sci.* 1984;7:223–268.
34. Nadel L, Hardt O. Update on memory systems and processes. *Neuropsychopharmacology.* 2011;36:251–273.
35. Cahill L, Babinsky R, Markowitsch HJ, McGaugh JL. The amygdala and emotional memory. *Nature.* 1995;377:295–296.
36. Hyman SE. A new image of fear and emotion. *Nature.* 1998; 393:417–418.
37. Iversen S, Kupfermann I, Kandel ER. Emotional states and feelings. In: Kandel ER, Schwartz J, Jessell TM, eds, *Principles of Neural Science.* New York, NY: McGraw-Hill; 2000:982–997.
38. Cahill L, Haier RJ, Fallon J, et al. Amygdala activity at encoding correlated with long-term, free recall of emotional information. *Proc Nat Acad Sci USA.* 1996;93:8016–8021.
39. Ullman MT. The role of memory systems in disorders of language. In: Stemmer B, Whitaker HA, eds, *Handbook of the Neuroscience of Language.* Oxford, UK: Academic Press; 2008:189–198.
40. Damasio AR. Aphasia. *N Engl J Med.* 1992;326:531–539.
41. Dronkers NF, Redfern BB, Knight RT. The neural architecture of language disorders. In: Gazzaniga MS, ed, *The New Cognitive Neurosciences.* Cambridge, MA: MIT Press; 2000:949–958.

42. Farah MJ, Grossman M. Semantic memory impairments. In: Feinberg TE, Farah MJ, eds, *Behavioral Neurology and Neuropsychology*. New York, NY: McGraw-Hill; 1997:473–477.
43. Ullman MT. Contributions of memory circuits to language: the declarative/procedural model. *Cognition*. 2004;92:231–270.
44. Damasio H, Grabowski TJ, Tranel D, Hichwa RD, Damasio AR. A neural basis for lexical retrieval. *Nature*. 1996;380:499–505.
45. Indefry P, Cutler A. Prelexical and lexical processing in listening. In: Gazzaniga MS, ed, *The Cognitive Neurosciences*. Cambridge, MA: MIT Press; 2004:759–774.
46. Martin A, Chao LL. Semantic memory and the brain: structure and processes. *Curr Opin Neurobiol*. 2001;11:194–201.
47. Ullman MT. The biocognition of the mental lexicon. In: Gaskell MG, ed, *The Oxford Handbook of Psycholinguistics*. Oxford, UK: Oxford University Press; 2007:268–286.
48. Mishkin M, Malamut B, Bachevalier J. Memories and habits: two neural systems. In: Lynch G, McGaugh J, Weinberger N, eds, *Neurobiology of Learning and Memory*. New York, NY: Guilford Press; 1984:65–77.
49. Mishkin M, Siegler B, Saunders RC, Malamut BJ. An animal model of global amnesia. In: Corkin S, Davis KL, Growdon JH, Usdin E, Wurtman RJ, eds, *Toward a Treatment of Alzheimer's Disease*. New York, NY: Raven Press; 1982:235–247.
50. Zola-Morgan S, Squire L, Mishkin M. The neuroanatomy of amnesia: amygdala-hippocampus versus temporal stem. *Science*. 1982;218:1337–1339.
51. Knowlton BJ, Mangels JA, Squire LR. A neostriatal habit learning system in humans. *Science*. 1996;273:1399–1402.
52. Bayles KA, Tomoeda CK. *Improving Function in Dementia and Other Cognitive-Linguistic Disorders*. Austin, TX: Pro-Ed; 1997.
53. Fodor, JA. *The Language of Thought*. New York, NY: Thomas Y. Crowell Company; 1975.

Unit 2

MCI: Minimal Cognitive Impairment

Alzheimer's disease (AD) begins insidiously and gathers momentum over many years before becoming clinically obvious.[1] Although no one knows exactly when the disease begins, some speculate that associated pathophysiologic processes begin a decade or more before individuals are formally diagnosed.[2] Because early identification is important to affected individuals interested in treatment and researchers investigating prevention, members of the National Institute on Aging and Alzheimer's Association workgroup[3] developed diagnostic criteria for presymptomatic as well as symptomatic AD. Presymptomatically, individuals can have evidence of *early pathological changes* but not meet clinical criteria for minimal cognitive impairment (MCI) or Alzheimer's dementia. Those with clinical evidence of early cognitive decline but who do not have dementia *meet the criteria for MCI*. The focus of this text is on the 2 clinically symptomatic stages: MCI and Alzheimer's dementia.

Mild Cognitive Impairment

MCI is a psychogeriatric syndrome with many causes that frequently evolves to frank dementia. The term *mild cognitive impairment* was first used by Flicker et al[4] to describe the cases of those individuals whose score on the Global Deterioration Scale was 3: not normal but not demented. The term has endured and is used to represent a cognitive state that is not the result of normal aging.

AD is the most common cause of MCI.[5] Other common causes include vascular disease, depression, Lewy body disease, and Parkinson's disease. Because MCI prevalence increases with age, and the elderly segment of the population is the fastest growing, clinicians and researchers worldwide are intensely interested in methodology for reliable early detection. Were an intervention available that delayed the onset of AD dementia by just 5 years, there would be a 57% reduction in the number of people with AD dementia and a reduction of $283 billion in Medicare costs.[3] Early detection affords affected individuals options that can slow or prevent development of dementia, among them pharmacologic and behavioral interventions and lifestyle change.

Whereas the effects of drugs used to treat clinically apparent AD are being evaluated for their potential to arrest disease progression in individuals with MCI, no drug has emerged as capable of preventing dementia, though some appear to improve cognitive function. What has emerged is evidence of the potential of cognitive stimulation for sustaining and improving information processing in individuals with MCI[6] (see Unit 6 by McCullough). Cognitive stimulation is noninvasive, cost effective, generally enjoyed by recipients, and free of the negative side effects of drugs. Speech-language pathologists are among those professionals qualified to screen for MCI and provide cognitive stimulation therapy to affected individuals.

Clinical Presentations of MCI

In 2003 an international conference was convened in Stockholm to consider the *clinical* characteristics of MCI. Conferees agreed that 4 subtypes are distinguishable (Table 2–1). A significant differentiating characteristic is memory impairment (present/absent); another is the number of cognitive domains affected (1 / >1).[7,8]

Although episodic memory impairment is known to be an early cognitive deficit in AD,[9] research and clinical experience have demonstrated exceptions. For example, neither the syndromes of posterior cortical atrophy[10] or logopenic-primary progressive aphasia[11] necessarily present with memory impairment but nonetheless can eventuate in AD. Posterior cortical atrophy typically manifests when individuals are in their 50s or early 60s and is characterized by problems with visual processing that reflect pathology in the back of the brain. Affected persons can have difficulty recognizing faces and objects or reading. In primary progressive aphasia, aphasia is the presenting symptom and persists for up to 2 years before memory and other cognitive impairment(s) are apparent.[12]

Table 2–1. Four Widely Recognized Subtypes of MCI

Amnestic MCI Single Domain	Subjective or proxy cognitive complaint; objective memory impairment; intact cognitive function; relatively intact functional ability; not demented.
Amnestic MCI Multiple Domain	Subjective or proxy cognitive complaint; objective impairment in memory and at least 1 other cognitive domain; intact cognitive function; relatively intact functional ability; not demented.
Nonamnestic MCI Single Domain	Subjective or proxy cognitive complaint; objective impairment in 1 nonmemory domain; intact cognitive function; relatively intact functional ability; not demented.
Nonamnestic MCI Multiple Domain	Subjective or proxy cognitive complaint; objective impairment in 2 or more nonmemory domains; intact cognitive function; relatively intact functional ability not demented.

Prevalence of MCI in the Population

Prevalence estimates of MCI vary considerably because of methodological differences in the age of study subjects (higher prevalence in older individuals), measures used to evaluate cognitive function, and the stringency of diagnostic criteria used. Nonetheless, results of a large community-based study of 2000 randomly recruited individuals between the ages of 70 and 89 indicate that the prevalence in the population approximates 16%.[13] Individuals with amnestic MCI are 2 to 3 times more common than those with nonamnestic. Prevalence is higher in men than women, people who never married, and those who carry 1 or 2 copies of the apolipoprotein (Apo) E4 allele. Also, its prevalence is related to years of education such that more years of education is associated with lower prevalence. As yet, however, the frequency of MCI subtypes has not been definitively established, although amnestic multidomain MCI appears to be the most common and amnestic single-domain MCI the least common.[14,15]

Diagnostic Criteria for MCI and AD

As previously noted, the collaborative efforts of the National Institute on Aging and the Alzheimer's Association resulted in recommended neurobehavioral and biomarker criteria for diagnosing MCI and AD.[16] The 4 *neurobehavioral* criteria that define MCI are:

1. *Concern regarding change in cognition compared with prior level*: Concern can be provided by the patient, an informant, or clinician.
2. *Impairment in 1 or more cognitive domains:* A performance in 1 or more cognitive areas (memory, executive function, attention, language and visuospatial skills) that is lower than expected for the patient's age and educational background. Most commonly seen is impairment in episodic memory. If repeated assessments are available, decline should be apparent.
3. *Preservation of independence in functional abilities:* Although individuals in the preclinical stage retain the ability to manage their daily affairs, they are less efficient doing so, make more errors, and require more time to task completion.
4. *Not demented:* The cognitive and behavioral changes are sufficiently mild as to fail to significantly interfere with social or occupational functioning.

Biomarkers are physiological, biochemical, and anatomic parameters that reflect the effects of disease-related pathophysiological processes.[17] Some markers indicate molecular neuropathology, such as the presence of signature proteins that accumulate in the brain during disease evolution; others include structural and functional changes, such as loss of hippocampal volume and reduction of glucose metabolism or perfusion in temporoparietal cortex that are revealed with positron emission tomography or single-photon emission computed tomography scanning. Yet other biomarkers indicate biochemical events such as inflammation.[17,18] Petersen and colleagues[13] reported that the majority of individuals with MCI have biomarker evidence of amyloid deposits or neurodegeneration or both. Abnormal levels of beta-amyloid are detectable early, brain degeneration is detectable later. Together with neurobehavioral changes, biomarkers increase physicians' confidence in making the diagnosis of MCI and predicting time to dementia conversion. They also provide researchers a standard method for characterizing subjects, thereby facilitating meta-analyses and results comparisons.

Conversion to Dementia

Individuals with MCI have elevated rates of conversion to dementia,[19] although considerable controversy exists about the percentage who will convert. Different investigators have used different criteria for defining MCI and used subjects who varied considerably in age. Those investigators who had more stringent diagnostic criteria (1.5 standard deviations below the mean performance of healthy age-mates on neuropsychological tests) had higher rates of conversion over shorter periods of time. Mitchell and Shiri-Feshki[20] analyzed 41 high-quality studies, some conducted on community populations, others on participants involved in clinical trials, and derived an annual conversion rate of ~5% to 10%. However, after 10 years, *more than half* the individuals originally diagnosed with MCI had not progressed to Alzheimer's or any other dementia. On the other hand, elders with MCI in the Mayo Alzheimer's Research Center study converted at a rate of 12% per year, and after 6 years, 80% had converted.[21]

Rates of *reversion to normal* vary in the literature. Ritchie et al[22] reported a rate of 15%, and Busse and colleagues 18% to 22%.[23] Improved cognition was most common in those with nonamnestic MCI. Also worth noting is that 4% to 13% of individuals diagnosed with MCI in the Busse et al study had a different diagnosis at follow-up evaluation.

Conversion Rate by MCI Subtype

As yet, the conversion rates by MCI subtypes have not been definitively established. A meta-analysis of results of conversion studies determined the rates to be 11.7% for amnestic MCI (9 studies), 12.2% for amnestic multidomain MCI (8 studies), and 4.1% for nonamnestic MCI.[20] With the new neurobehavioral and biomarker diagnostic criteria, more agreement among studies is expected. What is apparent, however, is that individuals with amnestic MCI are more likely to progress to dementia than those with nonamnestic MCI, and of individuals who convert, the large majority have AD.[24] In fact, a meta-analysis of results of longitudinal studies (average 3.1 years) of individuals with MCI showed that 90% of those who converted had the amnestic subtype.[5]

Some controversy surrounds the issue of whether a "pure amnestic" subtype of MCI exists. Several investigations have shown that comprehensive evaluation reveals other deficits, primarily in executive function.[25–27] Brandt and colleagues[26] administered 18 tests of executive function (spontaneous flexibility and generativity, inhibition of prepotent responses, planning and sequencing, concept/rule learning and set shifting, decision making and judgment, working memory and resource sharing) to 124 individuals with MCI who were subcategorized by subtype on the basis of screening tests and self-report. Deficits in the executive cognition domains of planning/problem solving and working memory were present in all 4 MCI subtype groups, although those with multidomain MCI had more executive problems than did those with single-domain. Albert et al[9] also observed that MCI patients who converted to dementia had lower executive function scores at baseline testing. Furthermore, the rate of change in executive function was greatest among those individuals who converted to dementia.

Number of Deficits and Conversion to Dementia

Simply stated, the greater the number of cognitive deficits, the greater the probability of conversion.[28] Hodges et al[29] conducted a longitudinal study of 10 individuals with MCI who were given extensive neuropsychological testing annually. All ultimately developed dementia (defined as <24 on the Mini-Mental State Examination [MMSE] and/or a significant problem with activities of daily living), although onset ranged from 1 to 8 years. Those who presented with multiple cognitive deficits early, including language, converted faster and were more likely to develop AD.[30,31]

Risk and Protective Factors

The most significant risk factor for MCI is age. The older the individual, the greater the probability. In a study of Americans, Petersen and colleagues (2006)[32] reported an MCI prevalence of 9% in individuals 70 to 79 years old and 18% in those 80 to 89 years old. APOE carrier status is another significant predictor. The ApoE gene is found on chromosome 19. It contains instructions for making a protein that transports cholesterol and other types of fat in the bloodstream. The specific composition of ApoE is influenced by the presence or absence of 3 major variants of the gene, which are called E2, E3, and E4. Individuals inherit a variant from each parent, most commonly ApoE3, which is carried by more than half the population. Individuals who carry the less common ApoE4 variant have a greater risk for developing MCI that will evolve to AD, especially if they have 2 copies.[33,34] Also, APOE carrier status has been associated with deficits in episodic memory and executive function.[9] Nonetheless, almost half the individuals with AD do not have the ApoE4 genotype, and the presence of an E4 allele accounts for a relatively small percentage of cases.[35,36] Other significant risk factors include diabetes, hyperlipidemia, current smoking, depression, high blood pressure, increased cholesterol, lack of exercise, high alcohol consumption, and infrequent social participation.[37]

Cognitive Deficits

By definition, individuals with MCI have cognitive deficits, and an extensive literature documents those associated with the various MCI subtypes.[26,27,38–40] Because language comprehension and production are subserved by cognitive processes such as memory, perception, speed of processing, attention, and various executive functions, it is unsurprising that *a strong correlation exists between scores on language measures and scores on measures of those cognitive functions needed to complete 1 or more language tasks.*[41]

Cognitive-Linguistic Deficits

Of significance to speech-language pathologists are the numerous reports in the literature that MCI is frequently associated with early impairment in language.[42] (See Taler and Phillips[43] for a review.) Indeed, language change in MCI is an area of intense research interest, spawned in large part from the now famous Nun Study.[44–46] Investigators had access to the autobiographies of almost 200 American

Roman Catholic nuns, members of the School Sisters of Notre Dame. Although the Nun Study began when the Sisters were between 75 and 103 years old, their autobiographies had been written decades earlier as novices. Linguistic analyses of their autobiographies revealed that nuns whose texts had lower idea density and grammatical complexity were more likely to develop AD later in life. Making this finding even more compelling was the similar life history of these nuns by virtue of their being in the same order, living under similar conditions, and the majority (85%) working as teachers. Since the report of Snowdon and colleagues, other investigators have also reported a relation between cognitive performance early in life and vulnerability to late-life dementia.[47,48] Though few investigators are able to compare the language performance of older subjects with their performance when they were young adults, many have included language testing in their studies of individuals at risk for MCI.[43]

An intriguing report of the sensitivity of language test scores for detecting MCI was published in 2009 by Oulahaj et al,[49] who followed a cohort of 241 normal healthy individuals for up to 20 years. The purpose of the study was to identify early markers of the later development of MCI. Subjects were periodically administered the Cambridge Cognitive Examination (CAMCOG), a widely used comprehensive neuropsychological battery comprising subtests of orientation, comprehension, expression, recent memory, remote memory, learning, abstract thinking, perception, praxis, attention, and calculation, as well as a derived MMSE score. Only the subscores for language expression and learning/memory were predictors of time to conversion to MCI. The CAMCOG expression subtest includes verbal fluency, spoken language descriptions, definitions, and comprehension. For each point lower on the CAMCOG expression score, the time to conversion was 17% shorter; for each point lower on the learning score, the time to conversion was 15% shorter; and for every 5 years of age, time to conversion was 14% shorter. The investigators emphasized that although memory impairment was the signature criterion of amnestic MCI and the recommended type of measure for assessing predementia AD, "expression" or language ability was a stronger predictor of duration to conversion than either "learning" or memory. It must be noted, however, that some would characterize verbal fluency as more a memory test than a language test. Nonetheless, it was just 1 of several language measures that formed the CAMCOG expression score.

Type of Language Changes

Various language deficits have been reported in naming and word retrieval, verbal fluency, language comprehension, discourse processing, and the ability to define words.[40,50]

Naming and Word Retrieval

Many investigators have compared the confrontation naming skills of individuals with MCI, those with mild AD, and healthy older adults and reported significant differences in the performance of those with MCI compared with healthy elders[51–53] and those with MCI and mild AD.[53,54] It is also the case that some investigators have failed to observe a significant different in confrontation naming ability of individuals with MCI and healthy elders.[22,55–58] Results differ because diagnostic criteria have differed, as have the lengths of the naming tests used. Perhaps the most important reason for differences is that only a segment of the MCI population has naming problems.

Saunders and Summers[27] compared individuals with subjective memory impairment (n = 32) with those with confirmed amnestic MCI (n = 60), mild AD (n = 14), and healthy age-mates (n = 25). All were given the Cambridge Automated Neuropsychological Assessment Battery (CANTAB), which is known to be sensitive to progressive declines in cognitive function over the course of AD. They were also given numerous other neuropsychological tests: the Wechsler Test of Adult Reading, the Dementia Rating Scale, the Boston Naming Test, the Rey Auditory Verbal Learning Test, and the Paired Associates Learning Test. Study results revealed that both the individuals with subjective memory impairment and those with amnestic MCI displayed impairment in language retrieval as well as in other cognitive functions. The language retrieval deficits were larger for the amnestic MCI group than for the subjective complaint group. Furthermore, all subjects with subjective memory complaint and 83% of those with amnestic MCI displayed impaired performance on at least 1 measure of attention or working memory, despite the fact that the Dementia Rating Scale–2[59] did not detect impairment in these areas. These data suggest that MCI classification criteria based exclusively on the presence of attention, initiation, construction, and conceptualization and memory (components of the Dementia Rating Scale–2) will exclude many aging adults who in fact have significant decline in other cognitive domains, among them language use. Furthermore, 35% of the subjects who had informant-corroborated memory decline did not display memory impairment but did display impaired attention or working memory deficits.

Verbal Fluency

Verbal fluency, also known as generative or category naming, has been widely studied in individuals using semantic and letter category naming tests. Verbal fluency tasks require examinees to generate exemplars of items in a category, such as animals or vegetables, or words beginning with a certain letter in a specified period of time, typically 1 minute. Examinees must remember the category while searching lexical or semantic memory. Cottingham and Hawkins[41] examined the relation between verbal fluency and memory test performance in individuals with MCI and hypothesized that there would be an association. They administered letter and semantic category tasks to 92 individuals with cognitive complaints referred for neuropsychological assessment by geriatricians. Study results indicated that increasing levels of memory impairment, as measured by performance on the Wechsler Memory Scale III, were accompanied by increasingly poorer performance in generating category items. Also, the verbal fluency scores of subjects were weaker than their reading scores, indicating the greater sensitivity of verbal fluency tests to cognitive decline.

An extensive literature documents deficits in MCI in both semantic and letter category naming, though semantic category naming is widely reported as more impaired.[29, 41 56, 60–69] Based on results of a meta-analysis of 153 studies of category naming[70] not only is semantic category naming more sensitive to early AD, it is more strongly correlated with verbal IQ.

Discourse Processing

In 2002, Chapman and colleagues[71] reported results of a study of 69 individuals (20 with MCI, 24 with mild AD, and 25 cognitively normal elders) who listened to a 578-word biographical narrative and then were asked to recount a "shortened version" that included the story gist. Subjects had a copy of the story to follow while listening to it being read. Thereafter, they had 5 minutes to study the story before giving a shortened version and answering questions about story details. Subject performance data revealed that both the MCI and AD subjects were impaired on all measures of "gist-level" processing and answering story details.

In 2005 the findings of the effects of early AD on the characteristics of the writings of a well-known author were published. Garrard et al[72] analyzed the text of 3 of Iris Murdoch's novels, one written early in her career in her 30s, a second written during her prime, and her final novel written a few years before her death from AD. Comparisons were made of the degree of lexical diversity in the 3 works. In Murdoch's last and least highly regarded work, vocabulary was more restricted and there were fewer unique word types relative to overall word count.

Harris et al[73] reported subtle changes in the discourse of 10 adults with MCI compared with 30 neurologically healthy young adults and 22 neurologically healthy older adults. Subjects were instructed to describe, in detail, activities associated with preparing for and taking a trip to New York City. They were advised to think about trip preparation, packing, and activities while there. A variety of discourse analyses were conducted: calculation of mean length of utterance, proportion of definite nouns, indefinite nouns, verbs and modifiers, and pronouns and mazed words (repetitions, false starts, reformulations, and self-corrections). Count was also made of the number of core concepts shared that were related to the story theme. Data analyses revealed that individuals with MCI provided less thematic information and more irrelevant comments and were more verbose than normal subjects. Significantly, performance on the discourse task was associated with performance on cognitive measures, including the MMSE.

In a related study, Fleming and Harris[74] sought to determine whether performance on the Trip to New York discourse task differentiated normal elders from 8 physician-diagnosed individuals with MCI in terms of discourse length, complexity, and quality using Systematic Analysis of Language Transcripts analysis.[75] Other analyses included counting the number of words and core elements plus calculating the average number of morphemes per T-units. MCI subjects produced significantly fewer words and core elements than control subjects, although the groups did not differ in average length of T-unit.

Summary

Impairment in language performance may be an early and telling manifestation of MCI. Results of studies of language performance in young and older individuals strongly suggest that language changes occur very early, perhaps decades before a clinical diagnosis is made, at a time when intervention would likely be most beneficial.

Summary of Important Points

- MCI is a psychogeriatric syndrome with many causes that frequently evolves to dementia.
- AD is the most common cause of MCI, with other causes including vascular disease, depression, Lewy body disease, and Parkinson's disease.
- There are 4 widely recognized subtypes of MCI: amnestic MCI single domain, amnestic MCI multiple domain, nonamnestic MCI single domain, and nonamnestic MCI multiple domain.
- Although not definitively established, it appears that amnestic multiple domain MCI is the most common, while single nonamnestic domain MCI is the least common.
- In a community-based study of 2,000 individuals, results indicate that the prevalence of MCI in individuals between the ages of 70 and 89 approximates 16%.
- The 4 neurobehavioral criteria that define MCI are: concern regarding change in cognition compared with prior level, demonstrated impairment in 1 or more cognitive domains, preservation of independence in functional abilities, and nondemented state.
- Individuals with MCI have elevated rates of conversion to dementia.
- The greater number of cognitive deficits an individual has, the greater the probability of conversion to MCI.
- The most significant risk factor for MCI is age.
- Individuals with MCI have cognitive deficits as well as deficits in linguistic function because language is a manifestation of cognition.
- Since the Nun Study, reported by Snowden and colleagues, other investigators have reported a relation between cognitive-linguistic performance early in life and vulnerability to late-life dementia.

■ Various language deficits have been reported in individuals with MCI, including: naming and word retrieval, verbal fluency, language comprehension, discourse processing, and the ability to define words.

References

1. Braak H, Thal DR, Ghebremedhin E, Del Tredici K. Stages of the pathologic process in Alzheimer disease: age categories from 1 to 100 years. *J Neuropathol Exp Neurol.* 2011;11:960–969.
2. Morris J. Early-stage and preclinical Alzheimer disease. *Alzh Dis Assoc Dis.* 2005;19:163–165.
3. Sperling RA, Aisen PS, Beckett LA, et al. Toward defining the preclinical stages of Alzheimer's disease: recommendations from the National Institute on Aging—Alzheimer's Association workgroups on diagnostic guidelines for Alzheimer's disease. *Alzh Dement.* 2011;7:280–292.
4. Flicker C, Ferris SH, Reisberg B. Mild cognitive impairment in the elderly: predictors of dementia. *Neurology.* 1991;41:1006–1009.
5. Bruscoli M, Lovestone S. Is MCI really just early dementia? A systematic review of conversion studies. *Int Psychogeriatr.* 2004;16:129–140.
6. Jean L, Bergeron M, Thivierge S, Simard M. Cognitive intervention program for individuals with mild cognitive impairment: systematic review of the literature. *Am J Geriatr Psych.* 2010;18:281–296.
7. Petersen RC. Mild cognitive impairment as a diagnostic entity. *J Intern Med.* 2004;256:183–194.
8. Winblad B, Palmer K, Kivipelto M, et al. Mild cognitive impairment—beyond controversies, towards a consensus: report of the international working group on mild cognitive impairment. *J Intern Med.* 2004;256:240–246.
9. Albert M, Moss MB, Blacker D, Tanzi R, McArdle JJ. Longitudinal change in cognitive performance among individuals with mild cognitive impairment. *Neuropsychology.* 2007;21:158–169.
10. Alladi S, Xuereb J, Bak T, et al. Focal cortical presentations of Alzheimer's disease. *Brain.* 2007;130:2636–2645.
11. Rabinovici GD, Jagust WJ, Furst AJ, et al. A beta amyloid and glucose metabolism in three variants of primary progressive aphasia. *Ann Neurol.* 2008;64:388–401.

12. Mesulam M, Weintraub S. Primary progressive aphasia and kindred disorders. *Handb Clin Neurol*. 2008;89:573–587.
13. Petersen RC, Roberts RO, Knopman DS, et al. Prevalence of mild cognitive impairment is higher in men: the Mayo Clinic Study of Aging. *Neurology*. 2010;75:889–897.
14. Sasaki M, Kodama C, Hidaka S, et al. Prevalence of four subtypes of mild cognitive impairment and APOE in a Japanese community. *Int J Geriatr Psych*. 2009;10:1119–1126.
15. Snitz B, Saxton J, Lopez O, et al. Identifying mild cognitive impairment at baseline in the ginkgo evaluation of memory (GEM) study. *Aging Ment Health*. 2009;13:171–182.
16. McKhann G, Knopman D, Chertkow H, et al. The diagnosis of dementia due to Alzheimer's disease: recommendations from the National Institute on Aging—Alzheimer's Association workgroups on diagnostic guidelines for Alzheimer's disease. *Alzh Dement*. 2011;7:263–269.
17. Jack Jr C, Albert M, Knopman D, et al. Introduction to the recommendations from the National Institute on Aging and the Alzheimer's Association workgroup on diagnostic guidelines for Alzheimer's disease. *Alzh Dement*. 2011;7:257–262.
18. Albert M, DeKosky S, Dickson D, et al. The diagnosis of mild cognitive impairment due to Alzheimer's disease: recommendations from the National Institute on Aging—Alzheimer's Association workgroups on diagnostic guidelines for Alzheimer's disease. *Alzh Dement*. 2011;7:270–279.
19. Summers MJ, Saunders NLJ. Neuropsychological measures predict decline to Alzheimer's dementia from mild cognitive impairment. *Neuropsychology*. 2012;26:498–508.
20. Mitchell AJ, Shiri-Feshki M. Rate of progression of mild cognitive impairment to dementia—meta-analysis of 41 robust inception cohort studies. *Acta Psychiatr Scand*. 2009;119:252–265.
21. Peterson RC, Morris JC. Clinical features. In: Peterson RC, ed, *Mild Cognitive Impairment: Aging to Alzheimer's Disease*. New York, NY: Oxford University Press; 2003:15–40.
22. Ritchie K, Artero S, Touchon J. Classification criteria for mild cognitive impairment: a population-based validation study. *Neurology*. 2001;56:37–42.
23. Busse A, Hensel A, Gühne U, Angermeyer MC, Riedel-Heller SG. Mild cognitive impairment: long-term course of four clinical subtypes. *Neurology*. 2006;67:2176–2185.
24. Visser PJ. *Predictors of Alzheimer Type Dementia in Subjects With Mild Cognitive Impairments*. Maastricht, Netherlands: Neuropsych Publishers; 2000.

25. Kramer JH, Nelson A, Johnson JK, et al. Multiple cognitive deficits in amnestic mild cognitive impairment. *Dement Geriatr Cogn Dis*. 2006;22:306–311.
26. Brandt J, Aretouli E, Neijstrom E, et al. Selectivity of executive function deficits in mild cognitive impairment. *Neuropsychology*. 2009;23:607–618.
27. Saunders NLJ, Summers MJ. Attention and working memory deficits in mild cognitive impairment. *J Clin Exp Neuropsych*. 2010;32:350–357.
28. Bozoki A, Giordani B, Heidebrink JL, Berent S, Foster NL. Mild cognitive impairments predict dementia in non-demented elderly patients with memory loss. *Arch Neurol*. 2001; 58:411–416.
29. Hodges JR, Erzinçlioğlu S, Patterson K. Evolution of cognitive deficits and conversion to dementia in patients with mild cognitive impairment: a very long-term follow-up study. *Dement Geriatr Cogn Dis*. 2006;21:380–391.
30. Alexopoulos P, Grimmer T, Perneczky R, Domes G, Kurz A. Progression to dementia in clinical subtypes of mild cognitive impairment. *Dement Geriatr Cogn Dis*. 2006;22:27–34.
31. Sacuiu S, Sjogren M, Johansson B, Gustafson D, Skoog I. Prodromal cognitive signs of dementia in 85 year olds using four sources of information. *Neurology*. 2005;65:1894–1900.
32. Petersen R, et al. Study presented April 4 at the American Academy of Neurology meeting in San Diego; 2006.
33. Aggarwal NT, Wilson RS, Beck TL, Bienias JL, Bennett DA. Mild cognitive impairment in different functional domains and incident Alzheimer's disease. *J Neurol Neurosurg Psychiatry*. 2005;76:1479–1484.
34. Tierney MC, Szalai JP, Snow WG, et al. A prospective study of the clinical utility of ApoE genotype in the prediction of outcome in patients with memory impairment. *Neurology*. 1996;46: 149–154.
35. Evans DA, Beckett LA, Field TS, et al. Apolipoprotein episilon 4 and incidence of Alzheimer disease in a community population of older persons. *JAMA*. 1997;277:822–824.
36. Myers RH, Schaefer EJ, Wilson PWF, et al. Apoliprotein E epsilon 4 association with dementia in a population-based study: the Framingham study. *Neurology*. 1996;46:673–677.
37. Etgen T, Sander D, Bickel H, Förstl H. Mild cognitive impairment and dementia: the importance of modifiable risk factors. *Deut Ärztebl Int*. 2011;108:743–750.
38. Storandt M. Cognitive deficits in the early stages of Alzheimer's disease. *Curr Dir Psych Sci*. 2008;17:198–202.

39. Storandt M, Grant EA, Miller JP, Morris JC. Longitudinal course and neuropathologic outcomes in original vs. revised MCI and pre-MCI. *Neurology*. 2006;67:467–473.
40. Twamley EW, Ropacki SAL, Bondi MA. Neuropsychological and neuroimaging changes in preclinical Alzheimer's disease. *J Int Neuropsych Soc*. 2006;12:707–735.
41. Cottingham ME, Hawkins KA. Verbal fluency deficits co-occur with memory deficits in geriatric patients at risk for dementia: implications for the concept of mild cognitive impairment. *Behav Neurol*. 2010;22:73–79.
42. Visser PJ. Diagnosis of predementia AD in a clinical setting. In: Richter RW, Zoeller-Richter B, eds, *Alzheimer's Disease. A Physician's Guide to Practical Management*. Totowa, NJ: Humana Press; 2003:157–164.
43. Taler V, Philips NA. Language performance in Alzheimer's disease and mild cognitive impairment: a comparative review. *J Clin Exp Neuropsych*. 2008;30:501–556.
44. Riley KP, Snowdon DA, Desrosiers MF, Markesbery WR. Early life linguistic ability, late life cognitive function, and neuropathology: findings from the Nun Study. *Neurobiol Aging*. 2005;26:341–347.
45. Snowdon DA, Kemper SJ, Mortimer JA, Greiner LH, Wekstein DR, Markesbery WR. Linguistic ability in early life and cognitive function and Alzheimer's disease in late life: findings from the Nun Study. *JAMA*. 1996;275:528–532.
46. Snowdon DA, Greiner LH, Markesbery WR. Linguistic ability in early life and the neuropathology of Alzheimer's disease and cerebrovascular disease: findings from the Nun Study. *Ann N Y Acad Sci*. 2000;903:34–38.
47. McGurn B, Deary IJ, Starr JM. Childhood cognitive ability and risk of late-onset Alzheimer and vascular dementia. *Neurology*. 2008;71:1051–1056.
48. Whalley LJ, Starr JM, Athawes R, Hunter D, Pattie A, Deary IJ. Childhood mental ability and dementia. *Neurology*. 2000;55:1455–1459.
49. Oulahaj A, Wilcock G, Smith AD, de Jager CA. Predicting the time of conversion to MCI in the elderly: role of verbal expression and learning. *Neurology*. 2009;73:1436–1442.
50. Cuetos F, Arango-Lasprilla JC, Uribe C, Valencia C, Lopera F. Linguistic changes in verbal expression: a preclinical marker of Alzheimer's disease. *J Int Neuropsych Soc*. 2007;13:433–439.
51. Dwolatzky R, Whitehead V, Doniger GM, et al. Validity of a

novel computerized cognitive battery for mild cognitive impairment. *BMC Geriatr.* 2003;3:4.

52. Grundman M, Petersen RC, Ferris SH, et al. Mild cognitive impairment can be distinguished from Alzheimer disease and normal aging for clinical trials. *Arch Neurol.* 2004;61:59–66.

53. Petersen RC, Smith GE, Waring SC, Ivnik RJ, Tangalos EG, Kokmen E. Mild cognitive impairment: clinical characterization and outcome. *Arch Neurol.* 1999;56:303–308.

54. Goldman WP, Price JO, Storandt M, et al. Absence of cognitive impairment or decline in preclinical Alzheimer's disease. *Neurology.* 2001;56:361–367.

55. Albert MS, Moss MB, Tanzi R, Jones K. Preclinical prediction of AD using neuropsychological tests. *J Int Neuropsych Soc.* 2001; 7:631–639.

56. Chen P, Ratcliff G, Belle SH, Cauley JA, DeKosky ST, Ganguli M. Patterns of cognitive decline in presymptomatic Alzheimer disease: a prospective community study. *Arch Gen Psych.* 2001;58:853–858.

57. Devanand DR, Folz M, Gorlyn M, Moeller JR, Stern Y. Questionable dementia: clinical course and predictors of outcome. *J Am Geriatr Soc.* 1997;45:321–328.

58. Schmidtke K, Hermeneit S. High rate of conversion to Alzheimer's disease in a cohort of amnestic MCI patients. *Int Psychogeriatr.* 2008;20:96–108.

59. Mattis S. *Dementia Rating Scale–2.* Lutz, FL: Psychological Assessment Resources; 2012.

60. Amieva H, Jacqmin-Gadda H, Orgogozo JM, et al. The 9 year cognitive decline before dementia of the Alzheimer type: a prospective population-based study. *Brain.* 2005;128:1093–1101.

61. Auriacombe S, Lechevallier N, Amieva H, Harston S, Raoux N, Dartigues JF. A longitudinal study of quantitative and qualitative features of category verbal fluency in incident Alzheimer's disease subjects: results from the PAQUID study. *Dement Geriatr Cogn Dis.* 2006;21:260–266.

62. Blackwell AD, Sahakian BJ, Vesey R, Semple JM, Robbins TW, Hodges JR. Detecting dementia: novel neuropsychological markers of preclinical Alzheimer's disease. *Dement Geriatr Cogn Dis.* 2004;17:42–48.

63. Fabrigoule C, Rouch I, Taberly A, et al. Cognitive processes in preclinical phase of dementia. *Brain.* 1998;121:135–141.

64. Grober E, Hall CB, Lipton RB, Zonderman AB, Resnick SM, Kawas C. Memory impairment, executive dysfunction, and

intellectual decline in preclinical Alzheimer's disease. *J Int Neuropsych Soc.* 2008;14:266–278.

65. Guarch J, Marcos T, Salamero M, Blesa R. Neuropsychological markers of dementia in patients with memory complaints. *Int J Geriatr Psychiatry.* 2004;19:352–358.

66. Hanninen T, Hallikainen M, Koivisto K, et al. A follow-up study of age-associated memory impairment: neuropsychological predictors of dementia. *J Am Geriatr Soc.* 1995;43:1212–1222.

67. Howieson DB, Carlson NE, Moore MM, et al. Trajectory of mild cognitive impairment onset. *J Int Neuropsych Soc.* 2008;14: 192–198.

68. Jorm AF, Masaki KH, Petrovitch H, Ross GW, White LR. Cognitive deficits 3 to 6 years before dementia onset in a population sample: the Honolulu-Asia aging study. *J Am Geriatr Soc.* 2005;53:452–455.

69. Nielsen H, Lolk A, Andersen K, Andersen J, Kragh-Sørensen P. Characteristics of elderly who develop Alzheimer's disease during the next two years—a neuropsychological study using CAMCOG. The Odense Study. *Int J Geriatr Psychiatry.* 1999; 14:957–963.

70. Henry JD, Crawford JR, Phillips LH. Verbal fluency performance in dementia of the Alzheimer's type: a meta-analysis. *Neuropsychologia.* 2004; 42: 1212–1222.

71. Chapman SB, Zientz J, Weiner M, Rosenberg R, Frawley W, & Burns MH. Discourse changes in early Alzheimer disease, mild cognitive impairment, and normal aging. *Alzheimer Disease and Associated Disorders.* 2002;16: 177–186.

72. Garrard P, Maloney LM, Hodges JR, Patterson K. The effects of very early Alzheimer's disease on the characteristics of writing by a renowned author. *Brain.* 2005;128:250–260.

73. Harris JL, Kiran S, Marquardt T, Fleming VB. Communication Wellness Check-Up©: age-related changes in communicative abilities. *Aphasiology.* 2008;22:813–825.

74. Fleming VB, Harris JL. Complex discourse production in mild cognitive impairment: detecting subtle changes. *Aphasiology.* 2008;22:729–740.

75. Miller J, Inglesias A. *Systematic Analysis of Language Transcripts (SALT)*, English and Spanish (version 9) [Computer software]. Language Analysis Lab, University of Wisconsin–Madison; 2006.

Unit 3

Alzheimer's Dementia

Alzheimer's Disease

Alzheimer's disease (AD) is the most common cause of dementia, and the number of affected individuals in the world population is near epidemic proportions,[1] more than 35 million people. Epidemiologists predict a doubling of patients every 20 years, thus by 2050 the number affected will soar to 115 million! AD is the sixth leading cause of death and the only cause among the top 10 that cannot be prevented or cured.[2] Each year there are 7.7 million new cases of dementia, or a new case every 4 seconds.

The cost of AD is staggering. In 2010 the cost worldwide was estimated to be US $604 billion, a figure that includes direct costs for medical care plus the cost of informal care provided by family and others.[3] If dementia care were a country, it would be the world's 18th largest economy; were it a company, it would be the world's largest, with annual revenue exceeding those of Wal-Mart ($414 billion) and Exxon Mobil ($311 billion).[3]

Diagnosing AD is challenging and is typically made by excluding other conditions associated with cognitive changes. Computed tomography (CT) and magnetic resonance imaging (MRI) are used to rule out tumor, cerebrovascular disease, and normal pressure hydrocephalus and to detect disease-associated atrophy in the medial temporal lobe and amygdalohippocampal system.[4] Increasingly, physicians are using biomarker data to make the diagnosis, and when paired with behavioral data, accuracy is high.

Diagnostic Criteria for AD

In 2011 a collaborative effort between the Alzheimer's Association and the National Institute on Aging resulted in revised diagnostic criteria.[5] The core criteria for *all-cause* dementia are cognitive and behavioral symptoms that: (1) interfere with the ability to function

Table 3–1. Overview of the Criteria for Probable Dementia

Probable AD	Impairment in 2 cognitive domains (language, visuospatial, executive or mood or behavioral symptoms)
	Evidence of progressive worsening of memory and other cognitive functions
	Insidious onset and clear history of worsening
	Absence of cerebrovascular disease or other neurological disorders that could affect cognition
	Symptoms cannot be explained by delirium or other major psychiatric disorder
	Biomarker evidence from MRI, PET, CSF increases certainty of disease as does evidence of a causative gene
Possible AD	Meets clinical criteria for AD but there is evidence of other systemic or neurological disorder that could affect cognition

at work or at usual activities, (2) represent a decline from previous levels of functioning, (3) are not explained by delirium or major psychiatric disease, and (4) represent cognitive or behavioral impairment involving at least 2 of the following: (a) inability to acquire and remember new information, (b) impaired reasoning and handling of complex tasks, (c) poor judgment impaired, (d) impaired visual spatial abilities, and (e) impaired language functions (changes in personality, behavior, or comportment).[6] Table 3–1 is an overview of the criteria for probable dementia.

Neuropathology of AD

AD affects the processes that sustain the health of neurons and ultimately destroys interneuronal communication. Historically, it was thought to begin in the cortex; however, recent evidence indicates that its genesis may be in the locus coeruleus,[7] a nucleus in the pons involved with homeostatic mechanisms. In a retrospective study, Braak and Del Tredici[7] observed "pretangle material" in the locus coeruleus in individuals under the age of 30. Over time the disease proliferates in perirhinal cortex (Figure 3–1), the hippocampal complex in the temporal lobes, and the basal forebrain, areas important to episodic memory.[8,9] Eventually, structural changes occur in the frontal, temporal, and parietal lobes. The brain areas most spared are motor and visual cortices,[10–12] a fact that accounts for the sparing of speech.

Motor symptoms can develop late in the disease, among them change in muscle tone, cogwheel phenomenon, postural instability, and difficulty walking. Collectively, these motor changes are referred to as "extrapyramidal signs,"[13] and their presence is associated with greater dementia severity.[14–18]

When tissue from the brain of an AD patient is examined microscopically, changes are apparent in the form of neuritic plaques, neurofibrillary tangles, atrophy, and areas of granulovacuolar degeneration. Deposits of amyloid within blood vessels may also be seen.

Neuritic plaques (Figure 3–2), called senile plaques in the older literature, are bits and pieces of degenerating neurons that clump together and have an amyloid core. Amyloid-beta is a protein fragment that has been separated from a larger protein called amyloid precursor protein. The disjoined amyloid-beta fragments aggregate and mix with other molecules, neurons, and nonnerve cells. Neuritic plaques are most prevalent in the outer half of the cortex, where the number of neuronal connections is largest.

Neurofibrillary tangles (see Figure 3–2) are disintegrating microtubules (microtubules are part of the internal support structure of healthy neurons). Microtubules disintegrate because of changes in tau protein that binds them in healthy brains, giving them supports. Tau is overphosphorylated in AD by enzymes that cause its detachment from the microtubules. As they disintegrate, they become tangled and are a signature morphologic change that confirms the presence of AD.

Atrophy, or the shrinking of tissue, is common in AD (Figures 3–3, 3–4, and 3–5), though it may not be visible on CT scan if the patient is in the early stage of the disease. Positron emission tomography (PET) scans show prominent changes in the temporal and parietal lobes and inconsistent changes in frontal lobes. MRI shows substantial atrophy in entorhinal cortex[19,20] and the hippocampal complex.[21,22]

Granulovacuolar degeneration refers to fluid-filled spaces within cells that contain granular debris.

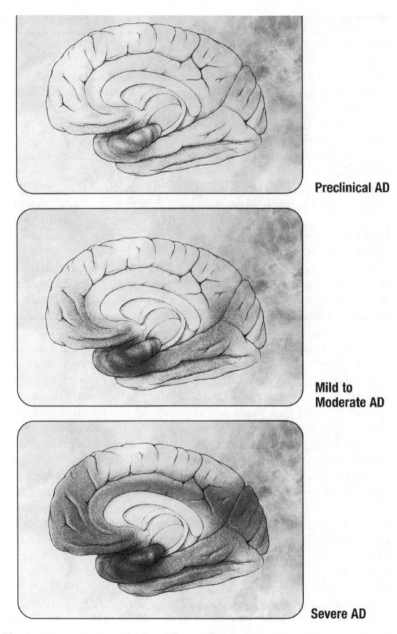

Preclinical AD

Mild to Moderate AD

Severe AD

Figure 3–1. Brain areas affected by Alzheimer's disease over the course of the condition. Darker shades indicate areas affected at the various stages of AD. From National Institute on Aging, *Alzheimer's Disease: Unraveling the Mystery.* Silver Spring, MD: Alzheimer's Disease Education and Referral (ADEAR) Center; 2002. NIH Publication 02-3782.

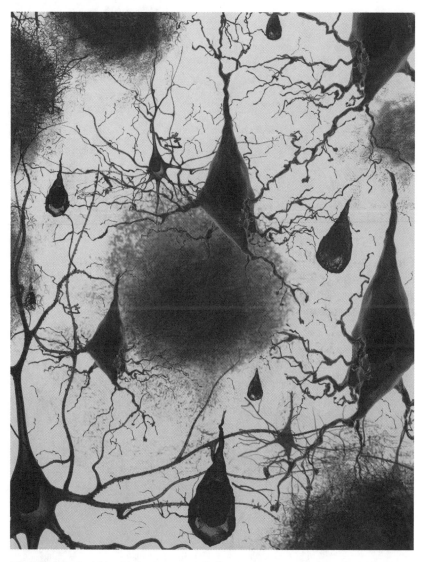

Figure 3–2. Neuritic plaques (center clump) and neurofibrillary tangles (Tadpole-shaped bodies). Image courtesy of *Alzheimer's Disease: Unraveling the Mystery*. National Institute on Aging/National Institutes of Health; 2008.

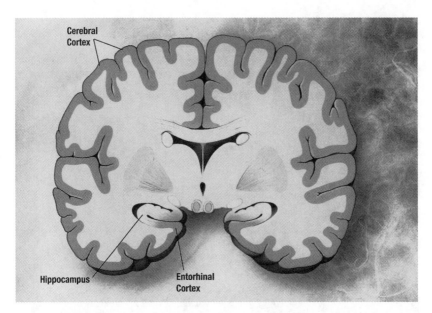

Figure 3–3. Schematic showing brain regions affected in the pre-clinical stage of AD. From National Institute on Aging, *Alzheimer's Disease: Unraveling the Mystery.* Silver Spring, MD: Alzheimer's Disease Education and Referral (ADEAR) Center; 2002. NIH Publication 02-3782.

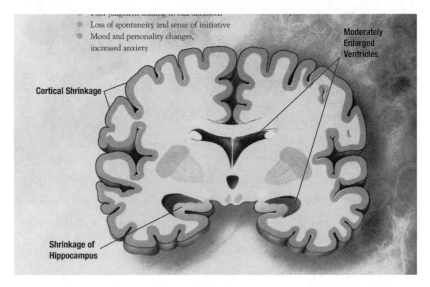

Figure 3–4. Schematic showing brain regions affected in mild AD. From National Institute on Aging, *Alzheimer's Disease: Unraveling the Mystery.* Silver Spring, MD: Alzheimer's Disease Education and Referral (ADEAR) Center; 2002. NIH Publication 02-3782.

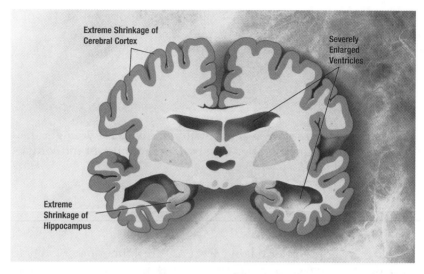

Figure 3–5. Schematic showing brain regions affected in severe AD. From National Institute on Aging, *Alzheimer's Disease: Unraveling the Mystery*. Silver Spring, MD: Alzheimer's Disease Education and Referral (ADEAR) Center; 2002. NIH Publication 02-3782.

Together these changes (neuritic plaques, neurofibrillary tangles, and granulovacuolar degeneration) in brain cells interrupt intercellular communication and thus information processing.

Risk Factors for AD

The following factors place an individual at increased risk for developing AD:

- Age
- Family history
- Less education
- Head trauma
- Loneliness
- Gender
- Age of mother at individual's birth

■ Having 2 copies of the type 4 allele of apolipoprotein E (ApoE4 allele)

■ Having minimal cognitive impairment (MCI).

Age

Clinically recognizable AD is unusual in individuals younger than 60, but for every decade after the sixth, the number of individuals with AD doubles.[23]

Family History of AD

People with a first-order relative with AD are 4 times more likely to develop it. However, the majority of cases are sporadic, with only 5% having familial/autosomal dominant inheritance. Familial AD often develops when individuals are in their 40s and is associated with a more fulminating course.[24–26] Results of twin studies indicate that when one twin develops AD, in only 35% to 50% of the cases will the other genetically identical twin be affected.[27]

Three genes are linked to early onset AD: the amyloid precursor protein gene on chromosome 21, the presenilin gene 1 on chromosome 14, and the presenilin gene 2 on chromosome 1. Note that the amyloid precursor protein gene is located on the same chromosome that is affected in Down syndrome, chromosome 21. The presenilin gene 1 on chromosome 14 is suspected of being responsible for the majority of early onset cases.

Definitions

Familial—occurring in more members of a family than would be expected by chance.

Autosomal—the gene is located on a chromosome other than the sex chromosome, so the disease is not sex linked; males and females are equally likely to be affected.

Dominant—the defective gene dominates its normal partner gene from the unaffected parent.

Less Education

Individuals with higher levels of education or IQ have been reported less likely to develop AD.[28–31] Uneducated individuals older than 75 have almost twice the risk for dementia compared with elders with 8 or more years of education. A popular explanation for this finding is that educated individuals have a richer network of interneuronal connections (and therefore greater cognitive reserve) that developed from the stimulation provided by more education.[32] Also, individuals with greater cognitive reserve may exhibit less impairment because they are better at mitigating cognitive loss through alternative strategies or compensations.

History of Head Trauma

Individuals with prior head injury may be at higher risk for AD.[30] Although the specific mechanism underlying the association of AD and head injury is not well understood, scientists theorize that head injury can alter the brain's protective system. Recently, researchers found head injury to be a risk factor for only those individuals with the ApoE4 allele.[33]

Loneliness

Loneliness is associated with greater risk for AD.[34] In a 4-year longitudinal study of the relation between loneliness/social isolation and presence of dementia, Wilson and colleagues[34] found that cognitive decline more than doubled in lonely persons compared with non-lonely individuals. However, in lonely individuals who died, loneliness was not associated with AD pathology or cerebral infarction, a result that suggests that loneliness may contribute to dementia risk through another mechanism. Wilson and colleagues suggested that the neural systems that support social behavior might be less elaborate in lonely individuals, making them less able to compensate for other neural systems being compromised by age and disease-related neuropathology. In fact, forced social isolation is well known to have a deleterious effect on the brains of animals.

Gender

Women have higher age-specific prevalence[35,36] and incidence[37,38] of AD than men. The gender effect remains to be explained, though some attribute it to the greater longevity of women.[39]

Maternal Age

Your mother's age at the time of your birth may influence your risk for developing AD. Both advanced[40] and early[41] maternal age have been reported as influential. The pathogenetic mechanism underlying the association of advanced or early maternal age and AD remains open for speculation.

Apolipoprotein E4 Allele

A type of cholesterol-carrying protein is a known risk factor for late-onset AD, namely, the ApoE4 allele. ApoE in the body varies in composition across individuals. The specific composition of ApoE is influenced by the presence or absence of 3 major variants of the gene: E2, E3, and E4. An individual inherits one gene that codes for the ApoE protein from each parent. The most common type is ApoE3, and most people inherit 1 or 2 copies. People who develop AD more commonly have the ApoE4 allele, and those with 2 copies of the ApoE4 gene have an 8 times greater risk for developing late-onset AD than individuals with no copies.[42] However, almost half the individuals with AD do not have the ApoE4 genotype, and the presence of an E4 allele accounts for a relatively small percentage of the cases of AD.[43,44]

Minimal Cognitive Impairment

Although MCI can have many causes, and the cognitive status of a significant percentage of affected individuals does not worsen, MCI can be an early manifestation of AD. Those with amnestic MCI are more likely to evolve to clinically apparent AD than those with the nonamnestic type.

Predictors of Disease Progression

The average duration of Alzheimer's disease is 8 years, though many victims suffer for 12 or more years. More rapid decline in AD is linked to:

- Early age at onset
- Presence of delusions or hallucinations
- Presence of extrapyramidal signs.

Protective Factors

Besides a higher level of education, a socially and cognitively active lifestyle later in life reduces the risk for AD.[45] So does regular physical exercise, which appears to have a neuroprotective effect.[46,47] A meta-analysis of 15 prospective studies of 33,816 individuals without dementia revealed that moderate and intense exercise reduced the risk for developing MCI by 35%.[48]

Effects of AD on Cognitive and Communicative Functions

As stated in the unit on MCI, the onset of AD is insidious, occurring many years before a clinical diagnosis is typically made.[49–52] Early neuropsychological deficits have been demonstrated by investigators using a variety of neuropsychological measures: psychomotor speed,[53] perceptual speed,[54] abstract reasoning,[55] visuospatial performance,[56] verbal ability,[57] and episodic memory.[50–52] Elias and colleagues[58] reported that lower scores on measures of memory and abstract reasoning were particularly strong predictors of probable AD.

The ever-present features of AD are impairment of episodic and working memory, especially executive functions. Other symptoms are more variable and reflect differences in the distribution of neuropathology.[59,60] Some patients have greater visuospatial than language deficits; for others, the reverse is true.[61,62] Those individuals with early-onset AD typically have less hippocampal involvement and greater atrophy in occipital and parietal cortices that results in poorer performance on visuospatial tests than memory tests.[63,64]

Results of longitudinal studies, using the Mini-Mental State Examination (MMSE), indicate that the average amount of cognitive decline per year is 2 to 4 points.[65] On the Alzheimer's Disease Assessment Scale–Cognitive (ADAS-COG), the average decline is 8 points per year.[16]

Early Stage

As previously stated, the pathophysiologic changes associated with AD begin years before behavioral and cognitive deficits are apparent. Thus, specifying the duration of the early stage is problematic. What is known, however, is the median age of survival after medical diagnosis of individuals in their 80s and 90s. Investigators in England followed more than 13 000 men and women, aged 65 and older, for 14 years.[66] In that period, 438 were diagnosed with dementia, most of whom died. Study results revealed that the men did not live as long as women: 4.1 years for men, 4.6 years for women. Frail individuals died earlier than those more physically fit. The investigators concluded that once an individual is medically diagnosed, life expectancy is approximately half that of a healthy individual of the same age.

When caregivers were asked to specify behavioral changes they observed before the diagnosis of AD was made,[67] they reported:

1. Difficulty handling finances
2. Memory problems
3. Concentration problems
4. Difficulty with complex tasks
5. Forgetting the location of objects
6. Decreased awareness of recent events.

Mental Status

In early-stage AD, the affected individual is disoriented for time but not place or person. Table 3–2 shows the average score, or range of scores, of early-stage AD patients on commonly used mental status tests.

Table 3–2. Average Score, or Range of Scores, of Early-Stage Alzheimer's Disease Patients on Commonly Used Mental Status Tests

ABCD Mental Status Test	7.3–12.5
Mini-Mental State Examination	16–24
Clinical Dementia Rating Scale	1
Global Deterioration Scale	3

Motor Function

Motor function is good and the patient is ambulatory.

Memory Function

The typical first symptom of AD is a problem with episodic memory: forgetting where the car is parked, getting lost, being repetitious, not remembering having taken medication, and the like. Working memory is also affected early and is manifested by decreased efficiency of encoding and retrieval of information. Individuals have difficulty sustaining attention,[68–71] and span memory is modestly attenuated in some individuals, though not all.

Basic Activities of Daily Living

Individuals in early-stage AD are generally able to carry out activities of daily living (ADLs), such as bathing, dressing, and feeding themselves and going to the bathroom independently.

Linguistic Communication

Speech is fluent in early AD, with no evidence of dysarthria or articulation errors.[72] Spoken language is grammatical, though errors of grammar and spelling are common in written language.[73,74] Content of language is noticeably affected and characterized by tangentiality and an increase in the number of "empty words" such as "thing" and "it." Because AD patients often forget what they just heard or thought, their oral discourse contains more sentence fragments and repetitiousness and is less cohesive than the discourse of healthy peers.[75–77] Then too, AD patients pause more frequently and have a slower speech rate.[78] Mild dysnomia is common, and when a naming error occurs, it is usually semantically related to the target word (eg, "lime" for "lemon," "sharp" for "saw").[79] Performances on tests of receptive vocabulary reveal that vocabulary is shrinking. Performance on tests of verbal fluency show significant deficits compared with healthy elders that worsen as the disease progresses.[71,80]

Language Use

Writing is more affected than oral language, and written discourse contains intrusions, perseverations, and more spatial-mechanical disturbances than that of healthy peers.[81–85] Although individuals in early-stage AD generally comprehend what they hear and read, they quickly forget it.[86] Mild AD patients often miss the point of a joke and may be confused by sarcasm. Some individuals exhibit logorrhea,[87,88] perhaps from disinhibition associated with frontal lobe damage. Early-stage patients are able to answer most questions and define words.[89]

Table 3–3 presents early linguistic communication symptoms,[90] listed in order of prevalence, from most to least frequent, as reported by 99 primary caregivers of AD patients. The most commonly reported symptom was word-finding difficulty. The least prevalent was an increase in talkativeness.

Discourse Sample of Mild AD Patient

The following discourse sample is typical of early-stage AD patients. The individual who produced this sample was instructed to explain what is happening in the Norman Rockwell painting *Easter Morning*. Rockwell portrays a man sitting in the family living room clad in pajamas and looking sheepish because he is not going to church with his wife and 3 children on Easter Sunday. Rather, he is staying home to read the newspaper, drink coffee, and smoke cigarettes. His wife and children are lined up behind him ready to go out the door.

It's evidently snowing outside of the window. And it's the mother I guess and the two girls and the boy, they are dressed like going to church. Because they each have Bibles in their hands. And this lazy goof. He sits in the chair and he's got his slipper this way and his eyes go over there. His hair looks like

Table 3–3. Linguistic Communication Symptoms Listed in Order of Prevalence from Most to Least Frequent (Bayles & Tomoeda[89])

Most Frequent
Word-finding problems
Difficulty naming objects
Difficulty writing a letter
Impaired comprehension of instructions
Difficulty sustaining a conversation
Problem completing sentences
Tendency to repeat ideas
Reading comprehension problems
Production of meaningless sentences
Decrease in talkativeness
Inappropriate topics
Inappropriate to whom said
Tendency to interpret literally
Failure to recognize humor
Increase in talkativeness
Least Frequent

hell. Pardon me. And whatever he's got on, it's ridiculous. And he, he, he is a good person to do that because he can do it. You know. Get his eyes over. And so, eh, he wants to stay home and see the funny papers and the newspapers and I love that Norman Rockwell anyway. And, eh, he's got his eyes almost out of sight. You know. But yet you can get him, he's a terrific guy. And so all these little darlings get to go to church. That's the way I see it because they each have a Bible their hand and, eh, he's looking to see what he can see. And it looks like he's saying, thank God I don't have to go. Eh, so that's about it.

Notice that the utterances are generally grammatical; however, compared with neurologically normal adults, this mild AD patient is a less efficient communicator. Also, she did not express the gist of the picture, namely that the wife is angry with her husband for staying home and he is feeling sheepish and guilty. The volume of discourse produced is not necessarily less than a healthy elder would produce but contains fewer ideas. Early-stage AD patients tend to repeat ideas, as did this woman, who repeated mention of the father's eyes, going to church, and holding Bibles. This phenomenon of *ideational perseveration* occurs more in mild and moderate patients than in severe because by the severe stage, individuals with AD have many fewer ideas.

Middle Stage

Many physicians and neuropsychologists define the middle stage by mental status. When individuals score below16 on the MMSE, they are recognized as being in the middle stage of the disease. However, no hard and fast rule exists for defining the difference between early and middle stage.

Mental Status

In midstage AD, the patient changes most dramatically, becoming increasingly dependent on others for survival. Disorientation worsens and includes confusion about place as well as time, although orientation to self is intact. Table 3–4 shows the average scores of midstage individuals on widely used mental status tests.

Motor Function

Motor function in midstage AD patients remains good, but restlessness is common.

Table 3–4. Average Score or Range of Scores of Individuals on Commonly Used Mental Status Tests

ABCD Mental Status Test	1.3–7.7
Mini-Mental State Examination	8–15
Clinical Dementia Rating Scale	2
Global Deterioration Scale	4–6

Memory

Many changes occur in memory in midstage AD, including worsening of episodic memory, attenuation of span memory, encoding and retrieval deficits, and degradation of semantic memory. Midstage patients have difficulty focusing attention, are easily distracted, and can be difficult to engage in activities. Visual-perceptual and visual-constructive deficits are apparent, and in fact AD patients perform inferiorly to healthy peers on virtually all executive function and cognitive-communicative tests.

Continence

During the later portion of midstage AD, incontinence of bladder becomes a problem.

Basic Activities of Daily Living

With supervision and environmental support, most midstage AD patients can carry out basic ADLs. In contrast, instrumental ADLs such as taking messages and managing finances are problematic. It is in this stage that driving becomes an issue. Although the midstage AD patient can manipulate the controls and mechanically drive a car, problems with attention, judgment, and memory make them dangerous to themselves and others.

Definitions

Activities of daily living—activities routinely performed in the course of an average day, such as feeding, bathing, dressing, and grooming.

Instrumental activities of daily living—activities related to independent living, such as preparing meals, managing finances, shopping, doing housework, and using the telephone.

Linguistic Communication

Speech. Speech is fluent, though often slower and halting and filled with more silent pauses that occur outside syntactic boundaries[78] and on more frequently occurring words.

Form of Language. The form of language remains generally intact but content is prominently affected.[86] Oral discourse contains fewer nouns relative to verbs,[73,91,92] is less cohesive,[93] and can be described as "empty." Performance on vocabulary tests indicates loss of vocabulary and greater degradation of conceptual knowledge.[77,86,94] Midstage AD patients are significantly impaired relative to healthy peers in generating exemplars of a category[95-98] and naming on confrontation.[86] Written language is replete with errors. Midstage patients exhibit diminished comprehension of written and spoken language,[99-104] although most do well at the word and phrase level. The mechanics of reading are spared but comprehension is impaired, and that which is comprehended is rapidly forgotten.

Language Use. Word-finding difficulties are now more obvious in spontaneous speech and on confrontation and generative naming tests.[72,95,105-107] Ideational repetition[76] is frequent in conversation and when individuals are asked to describe a picture or object. Midstage patients have poor sensitivity to context[108] and may miss the point of jokes. Also, they have a tendency to interpret nonliteral language literally. Although able to perform the mechanics of reading aloud, comprehend written language at the word level, and follow simple commands, midstage patients have serious difficulty defining words and repeating phrases.[89] In terms of writing, midstage patients make many spelling errors and mechanical distortions,[109] and their narratives are less complex.

Discourse Samples of Moderately Demented AD Patients

Sample 1: Task: Description of the *Easter Morning* picture

> Yeah, well, this man is, knows that he is, is in the wrong place here. So, but he's hiding away and, and these other people, I don't know whether this boy is ready to do it or not but this man is doing it from someplace over here, but it won't do it. And, ah, these, these, two children are evidently are just very excellent that they are both the same person. And, this man I don't know, would rather . . . He gets his too. And uh, oh, he's got this thing, worried because it's going to have a . . . going up there, you can see it. [Subject points to the cigarette smoke in the picture.] And all this stuff is just a mess.

Darn fools got anybody. Darn fools got them walking in it. They want to, I don't think they do. I don't want to go in this place. I don't know what he's for. He's looks like he's getting a ten paper. Here's some more paper. Here's some more, my god! Look at it. He has to be worn down before he can do anything, cause these people don't want to work, work anything with him. Don't you think that's about right?

Sample 2: Task: Individual is describing a marble.

Examiner: Tell me about this (marble).
Patient: Literally speaking, a marble. And the white is uh, is, uh, is the harder part. Well, it's a, I'd say cassium. The colored part, I don't know. Associated rocks. This is, uh, this is of the granitic nature. The whole thing. When you say cassium you're, you're talking about the hardest part of a, of a, of a rock. Well, there's some design to it. Some reason how it took that shape. But, uh, that doesn't mean a whole lot, exactly, the way someone de-, designed it.

As is apparent from these language samples, moderately demented AD patients produce discourse that expresses significantly fewer ideas than that of people with mild dementia. They are increasingly less concise and more repetitious. Intentions are often forgotten, resulting in many sentence fragments. As did the mildly demented patient, the individual who produced this discourse failed to state the gist of the Rockwell picture. The intention to describe remains, but word sequences often have little apparent meaning. Furthermore, there is a lack of self-monitoring and correction.

Late-Stage AD

During the late stage, AD patients often become disoriented for person as well as place and time. Their MMSE scores range from 0 to 9[110]; on the Clinical Dementia Rating Scale, they score 3.[111] Intellect is devastated by a global failure of working and declarative memory systems, and individuals are unable to carry out basic ADLs. There is incontinence of bladder and bowel. Motor impairment may be present, and in the very late stage, many are nonambulatory.

Linguistic Communication

Speech is typically fluent but generally slower and more halting. In many patients, the form of language remains intact,[112,113] although meaningful output is greatly reduced.[81] Some individuals are mute, others exhibit palilalia (repetition of phrases, words, or syllables that tend to increase in speed at the end of an utterance),[81] echolalia,[74] or jargon.[114] And yet, other advanced patients can contribute to a conversation, state their name, and retain aspects of social language.[115] Reading comprehension is severely impaired, although some can read single words aloud.[112,116] Virtually all late-stage patients are unable to express themselves in writing.

Communicative Abilities of Late-Stage AD Patients

The verbal communication abilities of 49 late-stage AD patients were evaluated in relation to other markers of late-stage AD (incontinence and ambulatory ability). The authors of 2 widely used tools, the Global Deterioration Scale[117] and the Functional Assessment Stages,[118] reported the *virtual loss of all verbal abilities in late-stage AD patients*. As part of a National Institutes of Health–supported longitudinal study of individuals with AD, Bayles and Tomoeda[116] were able to evaluate language in 49 late-stage patients. The Functional Linguistic Communication Inventory (FLCI)[116] was administered to these individuals. The FLCI evaluates greeting and naming, question answering, writing, sign comprehension and object-to-picture matching, word reading and comprehension, ability to reminisce, following of commands, pantomime, gesture, and conversation. Study results revealed that AD patients, who were *incontinent only for bladder*, had more communication skills than individuals who were *bladder and bowel* incontinent. They were able to respond appropriately to a greeting and to a closing comment and compliment. Several could recognize the written form of their name, state their spouse's name, recognize a common object from a line drawing, follow a 1-step command, and even correct misinformation about themselves.

None of the individuals who were incontinent for both bladder and bowel were able to contribute to a conversation. Neither could they state their spouse's name, follow a 2-step command, or provide relevant information about a common object. The most limited language was observed in individuals who were bowel and bladder incontinent and bedridden. However, contrary to what was expected, given previous characterizations of the verbal ability of late-stage patients,[118] *82% of the study participants produced language during the evaluation.*

The incontinent but ambulatory patients produced more words than those who were incontinent and nonambulatory. Of the 10 individuals who were incontinent but ambulatory, 1 AD participant produced 252 words and another produced a single word. Of the 17 individuals who were incontinent and nonambulatory, 3 individuals were nonverbal, 2 produced a single word, and 1 produced 131 words, of which 82 were different words.

The following are examples of answers provided by severely demented study participants to questions such as, "Where would you like to go on a trip?" and "What is your favorite food?"

"Right now I think I'd like to see Hawaii."
"Fruit of all kind is all right with me, I love fruit."
"I don't think I ought to go anywhere cause I'm in bad shape."
"I eat a lot of things now."

Discourse Samples of Severely Demented AD Patient

Sample 1: Task: Description of a button

Examiner: Tell me all about this [button].
Patient: Well, it's a button, with two holes in it for . . . for sewing on thread. That's the only . . .
Examiner: Can you tell me anything else?
Patient: Uh, that the only thing I can see.

Sample 2: Task: Description of a nail

Examiner: Tell me about this [nail].
Patient: That's a shingle nail. That's for tack on shingles and tack on roofing, and to tack on, uh, uh, its, er, a plasterboard.
Examiner: Can you describe it to me?
Patient: You mean this nail? Yeah, its long, short, small. That's uh, that about all . . .

As you can see, meaningful verbal output has diminished dramatically. However, grammar is generally intact. Without a context, listeners often have difficulty understanding what the AD patient is saying.

Summary of Important Points

- AD is the most common cause of dementia.
- The key diagnostic criterion for diagnosis is the presence of multiple cognitive deficits sufficient to interfere with social and occupational functioning that are gradual in onset and progressive in nature.
- AD begins in brain areas important to episodic memory and spreads to areas important to working and declarative memory. Procedural memory is spared until late in the disease course.
- The characteristic morphologic changes in the brain are neuritic plaques and neurofibrillary tangles, with areas of granulovacuolar degeneration and atrophy.
- AD rarely affects individuals younger than 60, but for every decade after the sixth, the number of individuals with AD doubles.
- A small number of individuals develop familial AD in their 40s, an autosomal dominant form of the disease.
- A type of cholesterol carrying protein has been found to be a major risk factor for late-onset AD, namely, the type 4 allele of apolipoprotein E.
- A diagnosis of AD reduces life expectancy to one half that for healthy age-mates.
- Communicative ability gradually deteriorates over the disease course. In the early stages, individuals are verbally fluent and able to comprehend most of what they read and hear but rapidly forget recently acquired information. By end-stage disease, individuals are intellectually devastated, and language output is greatly diminished and often nonsensical.
- Semantics and pragmatics are affected early; phonology and syntax are generally preserved well into the disease course.
- Considerable variability exists in the ability of late-stage AD patients to communicate. Some are mute, others produce some meaningful language.

References

1. Ferri CP, Prince M, Brayne C, et al. Global prevalence of dementia: a Delphi consensus study. *Lancet*. 2005;366:2112–2117.
2. Alzheimer's Association. Alzheimer's disease facts and figures. *Alzh Dement*. 2012;8:131–168.

3. Prince M, Bryce R, Ferri C. *The Benefits of Early Diagnosis and Intervention.* World Alzheimer Report. London, UK: Alzheimer's Disease International; 2011.
4. Knopman DS, DeKosky ST, Cummings JL, et al. Practice parameters: diagnosis of dementia (an evidence-based review). Report of the Quality Standards Subcommittee of the American Academy of Neurology. *Neurology.* 2001;56:1143–1153.
5. Lopez OL, McDade E, Riverol M, Becker JT. Evolution of the diagnostic criteria for degenerative and cognitive disorders. *Curr Opin Neurol.* 2011;24:532–541.
6. McKhann GM, Knopman DS, Chertkow H, et al. The diagnosis of dementia due to Alzheimer's disease: recommendations from the National Institute on Aging–Alzheimer's Association workgroups on diagnostic guidelines for Alzheimer's disease. *Alzh Dement.* 2011;7:263–269.
7. Braak H, Del Tredici K. The pathological process underlying Alzheimer's disease in individuals under thirty. *Acta Neuropathol.* 2011;121:171–181.
8. Braak H, Braak E, Bohl J. Staging of Alzheimer-related cortical destruction. *Eur Neurol.* 1993;33:403–408.
9. Van Hoesen G. Ventromedial temporal lobe anatomy, with comments on Alzheimer's disease and temporal injury. *J Neuropsych Clin Neurosci.* 1997;9:331–341.
10. Farkas T, Ferris SH, Wolf AP, et al. (18F) F2-deoxy-2-fluoro-D-glucose as a tracer in positron emission tomographic study of senile dementia. *Am J Psychiatry.* 1982;139:352–353.
11. Haxby JV, Grady CL, Koss E, et al. Longitudinal study of cerebral metabolic asymmetries and associated neuropsychological patterns in early dementia of the Alzheimer type. *Arch Neurol.* 1990;47:753–760.
12. Haxby J, Grady C, Duara R, Schlageter N, Berg G, Rapoport SI. Neocortical metabolic abnormalities precede non memory cognitive defects in early Alzheimer-type dementia. *Arch Neurol.* 1986;43:882–885.
13. Wilson RS, Bennet DA, Gilley DW, Beckett, LA, Schneider JA, Evans DA. Progression of parkinsonian signs in Alzheimer's disease. *Neurology.* 2000;54:1284–1289.
14. Mayeux R, Stern Y, Spanton S. Heterogeneity in dementia of the Alzheimer type: evidence of subgroups. *Neurology.* 1985;35:453–461.
15. Soininen H, Laulumaa B, Helkala EL, Hartikainen P, Riekkinen PJ. Extrapyramidal signs in Alzheimer's disease: a 3-year

follow-up study. *J Neural Transm Park Dis Dement Sect*. 1992;4: 107–119.

16. Stern RG, Mohs RC, Davidson M, et al. A longitudinal study of Alzheimer's disease: measurement, rate and predictors of cognitive deterioration. *Am J Psychiatry*. 1994;151:390–396.

17. Stern Y, Albert M, Brandt J, et al. Utility of extrapyramidal signs and psychosis as predictors of cognitive and functional decline, nursing home admission and death in Alzheimer's disease: prospective analyses from the Predictors Study. *Neurology*. 1994;44:2300–2307.

18. Stern Y, Mayeux R, Sano M, Hauser W. Predictors of disease course in patients with probable Alzheimer's disease. *Neurology*. 1987;37:1649–1653.

19. Krasuski JS, Alexander GE, Horwitz B, et al. Volumes of medial temporal lobe structures in patients with Alzheimer's disease and mild cognitive impairment (and in healthy controls). *Biol Psychiatry*. 1998;42:60–68.

20. Pearlson GD, Harris GJ, Powers RE, et al. Quantitative changes in mesial temporal volume, regional cerebral blood flow, and cognition in Alzheimer's disease. *Arch Gen Psychiatry*. 1992;49: 402–408.

21. Jack Jr CR, Petersen RC, O'Brien PC, Tangalos EG. MR-based hippocampal volumetry in diagnosis of Alzheimer's disease. *Neurology*. 1992;42:183–188.

22. Johnson SC, Saykin AJ, Flashman LA, Riordan HJ. Reduction of hippocampal formation in Alzheimer's disease and correlation with memory: a meta-analysis. *J Int Neuropsych Soc*. 1998;4:22.

23. Khachaturian ZS, Radebaugh TS. AD: Where are we now? Where are we going? *Alzh Dis Assoc Disord*. 1998;12(suppl 3): 24–28.

24. Jacobs D, Sano M, Marder K, Bell K. Age at onset of Alzheimer's disease: relation to pattern of cognitive dysfunction and rate of decline. *Neurology*. 1994;44:1215–1220.

25. Lovestone S. Early diagnosis and the clinical genetics of Alzheimer's disease. *J Neurol*. 1999;246:69–72.

26. Selkoe DJ. The genetics and molecular pathology of Alzheimer's disease: roles of amyloid and the presenilins. *Neurol Clin*. 2000;18:903–922.

27. Breitner JCS, Gatz M, Bergem ALM, et al. Use of twin cohorts for research in Alzheimer's disease. *Neurology*. 1993;43:261–267.

28. Katzman R. Education and the prevalence of dementia and Alzheimer's disease. *Neurology*. 1993;43:13–20.

29. Plassman BL, Welsh KA, Helms M, Brandt J, Page WF, Breitner JCS. Intelligence and education as predictors of cognitive state in late life: a 50-year follow-up. *Neurology.* 1995;45:1446–1450.
30. Kawas CH, Katzman R. Epidemiology of dementia and Alzheimer disease. In: Terry RD, Katzman R, Bick KL, Sisodia SS, eds, *Alzheimer Disease.* Philadelphia, PA: Lippincott Williams & Wilkins; 1999:95–116.
31. Sando SB, Melquist S, Cannon A, et al. Risk-reducing effect of education in Alzheimer's disease. *Int J Geriatr Psychiatry.* 2008; 23:1156–1162.
32. Stern Y. What is cognitive reserve? Theory and research application of the reserve concept. *J Int Neuropsych Soc.* 2002;8: 448–460.
33. Mayeux R, Ottman R, Maestre G, et al. Synergistic effects of traumatic head injury and apolipoprotein-E4 in patients with Alzheimer's disease. *Neurology.* 1995;45:555–557.
34. Wilson RS, Krueger KR, Arnold SE, et al. Loneliness and risk of Alzheimer disease. *Arch Gen Psychiatry.* 2007;64:234–240.
35. Hebert LE, Scherr PA, Beckett LA, et al. Age-specific incidence of Alzheimer's disease in a community population. *JAMA.* 1995; 273:1354–1359.
36. Schoenberg BS, Anderson DW, Haeren AF. Severe dementia: Prevalence and clinical features in a biracial US population. *Arch Neurol.* 1985;42:740–743.
37. Kokmen E, Chandra V, Shoenberg BS. Trends in incidence of dementing illness in Rochester, Minnesota, in three quinquennial periods, 1960–1974. *Neurology.* 1988;38:975–980.
38. McGonigal G, Thomas B, McQuade C, Starr JM, MacLennan WJ, Whalley LJ. Epidemiology of Alzheimer's presenile dementia in Scotland, 1974–88. *Br Med J.* 1993;306:680–683.
39. Jagger C, Clarke M, Stone A. Predictors of survival with Alzheimer's disease: a community-based study. *Psych Med.* 1995; 25:171–177.
40. Cohen D, Eisdorfer C, Leverenz J. Alzheimer's disease and maternal age. *J Am Geriatr Soc.* 1982;30:656–659.
41. van Duijn CM, Hofman A, Kay DWK. Risk factors for Alzheimer's disease: a collaborative re-analysis of case-control studies. *Int J Epidemiol.* 1991;20(suppl. 2):S1.
42. Corder EH, Saunders AM, Strittmatter WJ, et al. Gene dose of apolipoprotein E type 4 allele and the risk of Alzheimer's disease in late onset families. *Science.* 1993;261:921–923.
43. Evans DA, Beckett LA, Field TS, et al. Apolipoprotein epsilon-4

and incidence of Alzheimer disease in a community population of older persons. *JAMA*. 1997;277:822–824.

44. Myers RH, Schaefer EJ, Wilson PWF, et al. Apolipoprotein E epsilon 4 association with dementia in a population-based study: the Framingham study. *Neurology*. 1996;46:673–677.

45. Weuve J, Kang JH, Manson JE, Breteler MMB, Ware JH, Grodstein F. Physical activity including walking and cognitive function in older women. *JAMA*. 2004;292:1454–1461.

46. Etgen T, Sander D, Huntgeburth U, Poppert H, Förstl H, Bickel H. Physical activity and incident cognitive impairment in elderly persons: the INVADE study. *Arch Intern Med*. 2010;170: 186–193.

47. Singh-Manoux A, Hillsdon M, Brunner E, & Marmot M. Effects of physical activity on cognitive functioning in middle age: evidence from the Whitehall II prospective cohort study. *American Journal of Public Health*, 2005; 95: 2252–2258.

48. Pappolla MA, Bryant-Thomas TK, Herbert D, et al. Mild hypercholesterolemia is an early risk factor for the development of Alzheimer amyloid pathology. *Neurology*. 2003;61:199–205.

49. Braak H, Thal DR, Ghebremedhin E, Del Tredici K. Stages of the pathologic process in Alzheimer disease: age categories from 1 to 100 years. *J Neuropathol Exp Neurol*. 2011;11:960–969.

50. Collie A, Maruff P. The neuropsychology of preclinical Alzheimer's disease and mild cognitive impairment. *Neurosci Biobehav Rev*. 2000;24:365–374.

51. Grober E, Lipton R, Hall C, Crystal H. Memory impairment on free and cued selective reminding predicts dementia. *Neurology*. 2000;54:827–832.

52. Hodges J. The amnestic prodrome of Alzheimer's disease. *Brain*. 1998;121:1601–1602.

53. Masur DM, Sliwinski M, Lipton RB, Blau AD, Crystal HA. Neuropsychological prediction of dementia and the absence of dementia in healthy elderly persons. *Neurology*. 1994;44:1427–1432.

54. Rainville C, Fabrigoule C, Amieva H, Dartigues JF. Problem-solving deficits in patients with dementia of the Alzheimer's type on a Tower of London task. *Brain Cogn*. 1998;37:135.

55. Fabrigoule C, Lafont S, Letenneur L, Rouch I, Dartigues JF. WAIS similarities subtest performance as predictors of dementia in elderly community residents. *Brain Cogn*. 1996;30:323–326.

56. Howieson DB, Dame A, Camicioli R, Sexton G, Payami H, Kaye JA. Cognitive markers preceding Alzheimer's dementia in the healthy oldest old. *J Am Geriatr Soc*. 1997;45:584–589.

57. Jacobs D, Sano M, Dooneief G, Marder K. Neuropsychological detection and characterization of preclinical Alzheimer's disease. *Neurology*. 1995;45:957–962.
58. Elias MF, Beiser A, Wolf PA, Au R, White RF, D'Agostino RB. The preclinical phase of Alzheimer disease: a 22-year prospective study of the Framingham cohort. *Arch Neurol*. 2000;57: 808–813.
59. Galton C, Patterson K, Xuereb J, Hodges J. Atypical and typical presentations of Alzheimer's disease: a clinical neuropsychological, neuroimaging and pathological study of 13 cases. *Brain*. 2000;123:484–498.
60. Perry RJ, Hodges JR. Relationship between functional and neuropsychological performance in early Alzheimer disease. *Alzh Dis Assoc Disord*. 2000;14:1–10.
61. Fisher N, Rourke B, Bieliauskas L, Giordani B. Neuropsychological subgroups of patients with Alzheimer's disease. *J Clin Exp Neuropsych*. 1996;18:349–370.
62. Martin A, Brouwers P, Lalonde F, et al. Towards a behavioral typology of Alzheimer's patients. *J Clin Exp Neuropsych*. 1986; 8:594–610.
63. Frisoni GB, Pievani M, Testa C, et al. The topography of grey matter involvement in early and late onset Alzheimer's disease. *Brain*. 2007;130:720–730.
64. Fujimori M, Imamura T, Yamashita H, et al. Age at onset and visuocognitive disturbances in Alzheimer disease. *Alzh Dis Assoc Disord*. 1998;12:163–166.
65. Ballard C, O'Brien J, Morris CM, et al. The progression of cognitive impairment in dementia with Lewy bodies, vascular dementia and Alzheimer's disease. *Int J Geriatr Psychiatry*. 2001;16: 499–503.
66. Xie J, Brayne C, Matthews FE. Survival times in people with dementia: analysis from population based cohort study with 14 year follow-up. *Br Med J*. 2008;336:258–262.
67. Bayles KA. Alzheimer's disease symptoms: prevalence and order of appearance. *J Appl Gerontol*. 1991;10:419–430.
68. Bäckman L, Small BJ, Fratiglioni L. Stability of the preclinical episodic memory deficit in Alzheimer's disease. *Brain*. 2001;124: 96–102.
69. Grady C, Haxby J, Horwitz B, et al. Longitudinal study of the early neuropsychological and cerebral metabolic changes in dementia of the Alzheimer type. *J Clin Exp Neuropsych*. 1988;10: 576–596.

70. Morris RGM. Attentional and executive dysfunction. In: Morris RGM, ed, *The Cognitive Neuropsychology of Alzheimer-type Dementia*. New York, NY: Oxford University Press; 1996:49–70.
71. Perry R, Watson P, Hodges J. The nature and staging of attention dysfunction in early (minimal and mild) Alzheimer's disease: relationship to episodic and semantic memory impairment. *Neuropsychologia*. 2000;38:252–271.
72. Weiner MF, Neubecker KE, Bret ME, Hynan LS. Language in Alzheimer's disease. *J Clin Psychiatry*. 2008;69:1223–1227.
73. Blanken G, Dittmann J, Haas J, Wallesch C. Spontaneous speech in senile dementia and aphasia: implications for a neurolinguistic model of language production. *Cognition*. 1987;27:247–274.
74. Irigaray L. Approche psycho-linguistique du langage des dements. *Neuropsychologia*. 1967;5:25–52.
75. Bayles KA, Tomoeda CK, Boone DR. A view of age-related changes in language function. *Dev Neuropsych*. 1985;1:231–264.
76. Bayles KA, Tomoeda CK, Kaszniak AW, Stern LZ, Eagans KK. Patterns of perseveration of dementia patients. *Brain Lang*. 1985; 25:102–116.
77. Tomoeda CK, Bayles, KA. Longitudinal effects of Alzheimer's disease on discourse production. *Alzh Dis Assoc Disord*. 1993;7: 223–236.
78. Gayraud F, Lee H-R, Barkat-Defradas M. Syntactic and lexical context of pauses and hesitations in the discourse of Alzheimer's patients and healthy elderly subjects. *Clin Ling Phon*. 2011;25: 198–209.
79. Bayles KA, Tomoeda CK. Confrontation naming impairment in dementia. *Brain Lang*. 1983;19:98–114.
80. Small BJ, Bäckman L. Predictors of longitudinal changes in memory, visuospatial, and verbal functioning in very old demented adults. *Dement Geriatr Cogn Disord*. 1998;9:258–266.
81. Appell J, Kertesz A, Fisman M. A study of language functioning in Alzheimer's patients. *Brain Lang*. 1982;17:73–91.
82. Croisile B. Agraphia in Alzheimer's disease. *Dement Geriatr Cogn Disord*. 1999;10:226–230.
83. Groves-Wright K, Neils-Strunjas J, Burnett R, O'Neill MJ. A comparison of verbal and written language in Alzheimer's disease. *J Comm Disord*. 2004;37:109–130.
84. Horner J, Heyman A, Dawson D, Rogers H. The relationship of agraphia to the severity of dementia in Alzheimer's disease. *Arch Neurol*. 1988;45:760–763.

85. Kertesz A, Appell J, Fisman M. The dissolution of language in Alzheimer's disease. *Can J Neurol Sci.* 1986;13:415–418.
86. Bayles KA, Tomoeda CK, Trosset MW. Relation of linguistic communication abilities of Alzheimer's patients to stage of disease. *Brain Lang.* 1992;42:454–472.
87. Gustafson L, Hagberg B, Ingvar D. Speech disturbances in presenile dementia related to local cerebral blood flow abnormalities in the dominant hemisphere. *Brain Lang.* 1978;5:103–118.
88. Obler LK, Albert ML. Historical notes: Jules Séglas on language in dementia. *Brain Lang.* 1985;24:314–325.
89. Bayles KA, Tomoeda CK. *Arizona Battery for Communication Disorders of Dementia.* Austin, TX: Pro-Ed; 1993.
90. Bayles KA, Tomoeda CK. Caregiver report of prevalence and appearance order of linguistic symptoms in Alzheimer's patients. *Gerontologist.* 1991;31:210–216.
91. Fung T, Chertkow H, Templeman F. Pattern of semantic memory impairment in dementia of Alzheimer's type. *Brain Cogn.* 2000; 43:200–205.
92. Robinson G, Rossor M, Cipolotti L. Selective sparing of verb naming in a case of severe Alzheimer's disease. *Cortex.* 1999;35: 443–450.
93. Critchley M. The neurology of psychotic speech. *Brit J Psychiatry.* 1964;110:353–364.
94. Hier D, Hagenlocker K, Shindler A. Language disintegration in dementia: effects of etiology and severity. *Brain Lang.* 1985; 25:117–133.
95. Bayles KA, Tomoeda CK. Confrontation naming and generative naming abilities of dementia patients. In: Brookshire R, ed, *Clinical Aphasiology Conference Proceedings 1983.* Minneapolis, MN: BRK Publications; 1983b:304–315.
96. Bayles KA, Salmon DP, Tomoeda CK, et al. Semantic and letter category naming in Alzheimer's patients: a predictable difference. *Dev Neuropsych.* 1989;5:335–347.
97. Hodges J, Salmon D, Butters N. Differential impairment of semantic and episodic memory in Alzheimer's and Huntington's diseases: a controlled prospective study. *J Neurol Neurosurg Psychiatry.* 1990;53:1089–1095.
98. Huff F, Corkin S, Growdon J. Semantic impairment and anomia in Alzheimer's disease. *Brain Lang.* 1986;28:235–249.
99. Bayles KA. Language function in senile dementia. *Brain Lang.* 1982;16:265–280.

100. Cummings J, Benson F, Hill M, Read S. Aphasia in dementia of the Alzheimer type. *Neurology.* 1985;35:394–397.
101. Faber-Langendoen K, Morris JC, Knesevich JW, LaBarge E, Miller JP, Berg L. Aphasia in senile dementia of the Alzheimer type. *Ann Neurol.* 1998;23:365–370.
102. Horner J, Dawson D, Heyman A, McGorman-Fish A. The usefulness of the Western Aphasia Battery for differential diagnosis of Alzheimer dementia and focal stroke syndromes: preliminary evidence. *Brain Lang.* 1992;42:77–88.
103. Kempler D, Almor A, Tyler L, Andersen E, MacDonald M. Sentence comprehension deficits in Alzheimer's disease: a comparison of off-line vs. on-line sentence processing. *Brain Lang.* 1998;64:297–316.
104. Rochon E, Waters GS, Caplan D. The relationship between measures of working memory and sentence comprehension in patients with Alzheimer's disease. *J Speech Lang Hear Res.* 2000;43:395–413.
105. Benson DF. Neurologic correlates of anomia. In: Whitaker H, Whitaker HA, eds, *Studies in Neurolinguistics* (vol 4). New York, NY: Academic Press; 1979:298–328.
106. Kirshner H, Webb W, Kelly M. The naming disorder of dementia. *Neuropsychologia.* 1984;22:23–30.
107. Salmon D, Butters N, Chan A. The deterioration of semantic memory in Alzheimer's disease. *Can J Exp Psych.* 1999;53:108–116.
108. Tomoeda CK, Bayles KA, Trosset MW, Azuma T, McGeagh A. Cross-sectional analysis of Alzheimer disease effects on oral discourse in a picture description task. *Alzh Dis Assoc Disord.* 1996;10:204–215.
109. Neils-Strunjas J, Groves-Wright K, Mashima P, Harnish S. Dysgraphia in Alzheimer's disease: a review for clinical and research purposes. *J Speech Lang Hear Res.* 2006;49:1313–1330.
110. Folstein MF, Folstein SE, McHugh PR. "Mini-Mental State": a practical method for grading the mental state of patients for the clinician. *J Psychiatric Res.* 1975;12:189–198.
111. Hughes CP, Berg L, Danziger WL, Coben LA, Martin RL. A new clinical scale for the staging of dementia. *Brit J Psychiatry.* 1982;140:566–572.
112. Bayles KA, Tomoeda CK, Cruz RF, Mahendra N. Communication abilities of individuals with late-stage Alzheimer's disease. *Alzh Dis Assoc Disord.* 2000;14:176–181.

113. Mayhew PA, Acton GJ, Yauk S, Hopkins BA. Communication from individuals with advanced DAT: can it provide clues to their sense of self-awareness and well-being. *Geriatr Nurs*. 2001; 22:106–110.
114. Obler LK, Albert ML. Language in aging. In: Albert ML, ed, *Clinical Neurology of Aging*. New York, NY: Oxford University Press; 1984:245–252.
115. Kim ES, Bayles KA. Communication in late-stage Alzheimer's disease: relation to functional markers of disease severity. *Alzh Care Quarterly*. 2007;8:43–52.
116. Bayles KA, Tomoeda CK. *Functional Linguistic Communication Inventory*. Austin, TX: Pro-Ed; 1994.
117. Reisberg B, Ferris SH, de Leon MJ, Crooke T. The global deterioration scale for assessment of primary degenerative dementia. *Am J Psychiatry*. 1982;139:1136–1139.
118. Reisberg G, Ferris SH, Anand R, et al. Functional staging of dementia of the Alzheimer type. *Ann N Y Acad Sci*. 1984;435: 481–483.

Unit 4

Assessment of Cognitive-Communicative Function in Minimal Cognitive Impairment and Alzheimer's Dementia

The purpose of this unit is to explain procedures and tests used in assessing cognitive-communicative functioning in individuals at risk for minimal cognitive impairment (MCI) and those with Alzheimer's dementia (AD). The unit is organized such that assessment procedures common to both conditions are covered first, followed by assessment of individuals with MCI and those with clinically apparent AD.

Role of the Speech-Language Pathologist

The position of the American Speech-Language-Hearing Association (ASHA) is that speech-language pathologists (SLPs) play a primary role in the screening, assessment, diagnosis, and treatment of cognitive-communicative disorders, including those associated with dementing diseases. Additionally, ASHA recommends that SLPs identify persons at risk for dementia.

The Process of Assessment

The diagnosis of MCI or AD is made on the basis of history, performance on neuropsychological tests, perceptions of patients and families, and laboratory and imaging results. Assessment of cognitive-communicative function provides valuable information in making a diagnosis and allows clinicians to:

- Detect the clinical features of MCI or AD
- Characterize cognitive-communicative function
- Establish a baseline of cognitive-communicative functioning for designing treatment and measuring response to treatment
- Counsel caregivers
- Predict skills vulnerable to future decline.

Prior to Testing

Review Medical History

Clinicians should review the patient's medical history for information about possible sensory impairments (eg, macular degeneration, moderate to severe hearing loss) or other conditions that can alter cognitive functioning (eg, depression, medications). Also, they should determine the patient's level of education. If the patient was previously diagnosed as having probable AD, then severity of dementia may be specified in the record. Table 4–1 contains a brief description of commonly used rating scales of dementia severity and the scores that correspond to mild, moderate, and severe dementia. The patient's ability to see, hear, and read printed materials, as well as a description of the presenting symptoms and progression, can be verified by interviewing an informed caregiver prior to the assessment.

Secure a Quiet, Well-Lit Test Environment

Arrange for testing to take place in a quiet room with adequate lighting. The examiner should ensure that no shadows are cast on test materials and all stimuli are visible. Also, glare can impair an

Table 4–1. Three Commonly Used Measures of Dementia Severity and Scores/Ratings That Correspond to Mild, Moderate, and Severe Dementia

Measure	Mild Dementia	Moderate Dementia	Severe Dementia
Global Deterioration Scale (GDS).[74] The course of dementia is defined in 7 stages that have specific observational criteria. GDS stage 1 represents "normal" aging without evidence of cognitive decline. GDS stage 7 represents "late dementia" with very severe cognitive decline.	3 or 4	5 or 7	7
Clinical Dementia Rating Scale (CDR).[80] The CDR provides a rating of global cognitive function based on clinical information about memory, orientation, judgment, problem-solving, community affairs, home and hobbies, and personal care. Level of impairment is rated as none (0), questionable (0.5), mild (1), moderate (2), or severe (3).	CDR 1	CDR 2	CDR 3
Dementia Rating Scale (DRS).[81] The DRS contains items that evaluate five cognitive functions: attention, initiation and perseveration, construction, conceptualization, and memory. A maximum of 144 points can be awarded, and normal elders obtain scores of 140 or more.	120–130	90–119	< 90

73

elder's vision. If the examiner's back is to a bright light or window, the examinee will have difficulty seeing the examiner's face.

Testing

Check Vision

Visual acuity diminishes with age, and many elders need glasses to read. Make sure the patient wears eyeglasses if they are needed. If a patient's visual acuity is unknown, ask the patient to read simple words in a print size smaller than the test stimuli. If the patient can read text in the smaller print, then the examiner can infer that the patient has adequate visual acuity to see the printed test material. The examiner also can check for the presence of visual field deficits by administering a simple letter cancellation task such as provided in the Arizona Battery of Communication Disorders of Dementia, the ABCD.[1]

Check Hearing

Hearing loss becomes more common with age.[2,3] If the patient has hearing aids, make sure the patient wears them during testing. If the patient's hearing status cannot be determined, the examiner can administer a simple speech discrimination test to ensure that the examiner's voice is audible in the test setting. A speech discrimination task, in which the examinee is asked to repeat words that are the same or sound similar (like "map" and "lap"), can be found in the ABCD.[1] An error rate of 30% or greater indicates that the patient's hearing will likely impact test performance.

Check Literacy

If information about the patient's premorbid ability to read and write cannot be obtained, then the examiner should have the patient read 2 or 3 simple sentences aloud. Even individuals with moderate to severe dementia are able to read aloud if they were literate prior to the onset of cognitive symptoms.

Be Alert to Depression

Depression is more common in older adults and can be mistaken for dementia because it negatively affects test performance. When this occurs, the individual is said to have pseudodementia. Depression also frequently accompanies Alzheimer's and other diseases associated with dementia, such as Parkinson's. Thus, clinicians need to be alert to behaviors that suggest depression, among them:

Statements about feeling sad or helpless

Self-deprecatory comments

Disinterest in the testing and its outcome

Monotone voice

Low volume

Slow speaking rate

Lethargy

Inattentiveness

Indecisiveness

Inconsistency in performance.

A particularly important sign of depression is inconsistency in performance. Depressed individuals often perform better than would be expected on hard tasks if they have dementia, and poorer than would be expected on easy tasks. Because elders typically perform better earlier in the day, clinicians should take into account a possible effect on performance from the time of day the tests are given. Clinicians can screen for depression and refer those at risk to professionals qualified in depression treatment. Table 4–2 contains a brief description of commonly used measures. Some are interviewer administered and others are self-administered. For elders with cognitive deficits, interviewer-administered instruments are more appropriate.[4]

Be Alert to Adverse Drug Effects on Performance

Typically, the elderly take multiple medications to manage chronic diseases associated with aging.[5] The potential for adverse drug

Table 4–2. Tests That Can Be Used to Screen for Depression in the Elderly

Name of Measure	Citation	Description
Hamilton Rating Scale for Depression (HRS-D)	Hamilton, 1967[82] Hamilton, 1970[83]	The HRS-D is one of the first developed and best-known interview-based rating scales for depression. It is a 17-item inventory of symptoms that are rated for severity by an experienced clinician, based upon interview and other available data.
Beck Depression Inventory	Beck et al, 1961[84]	The BDI is a 21-item inventory of depressive symptoms and attitudes that are rated from 0 to 3 in terms of intensity. The BDI is commonly used as a self-administered measure, although it was designed for administration by trained interviewers.
Zung Self-Rating Depression Scales (SDS)	Zung, 1965[85]	The SDS comprises 20 items that evaluate four areas of disturbance: pervasive psychic, physiological, psychomotor, and psychological. The patient rates the applicability, within the past week, of each item according to the following terms: "none or a little of the time," "some of the time," "good part of the time," and "most or all of the time."

Zung Depression Status Inventory (DSI)	Zung, 1972[86]	The 20 items of the DSI correspond to the SDS, however, the interviewer rates the severity of symptoms or signs on a 4-point scale from none to severe based on the results of a clinical interview.
Dementia Mood Assessment Scale	Sunderland et al., 1988[87]	This two-part instrument is designed to measure the severity of mood disturbance of demented patients based on direct observation and a semistructured interview by health professionals. The first 17 items evaluate mood and are scaled from 0 (within normal limits) to 6 (most severe). The remaining seven items measure the patient's functional capacities.
Cornell Scale for Depression in Dementia	Alexopoulus, Abrams, Young, & Shamoian, 1988[88]	The Cornell Scale is a 19-item clinician administered instrument that uses information obtained from interviews with the patient and a member of the nursing staff. This instrument was specifically designed for measuring depression in demented patients.

interactions increases with advancing age and as the number of prescribed medications increases.[6] Sloan[7] reported that the potential for drug interaction is 5.6% when patients are taking 2 drugs and increases to 100% when patients are taking 8 or more drugs. Similarly, Larson and colleagues[8] found that drug reactions that impair cognitive function increase as the number of prescription drugs increases. In a review of 32 studies in which the prevalence of various causes of dementia was examined, Clarfield[9] reported that a common cause of reversible dementia was drug side effects.

Be aware that elders taking multiple medications are at higher risk for impaired mental status as a result of drugs. According to Orange,[10] the classes of drugs that commonly interfere with speech, language, and cognition are sedatives, antidepressants, anxiolytics (antianxiety drugs), antipsychotics, anticoagulants, antihypertensives, and narcotic-based analgesics. Sedative hypnotic agents, especially long-acting benzodiazepines, are the drugs most strongly associated with cognitive impairment.

Use Appropriate Tests

Efforts to refine the criteria for identifying individuals in the various stages of AD (asymptomatic preclinical, symptomatic predementia, and clinically apparent) are ongoing.[11–13] The National Institutes of Health–Alzheimer's Disease and Related Disorders Association working group acknowledges that definitive points at which individuals transition from one phase to another are difficult to specify. Consequently it proposes a model in which the pathophysiological sequence of AD leads to greater cognitive impairment, a so-called pathological-clinical continuum of AD.[13]

We have found, and others have confirmed,[14] that tests suitable for early detection of cognitive impairment are unsuitable for documenting decline of abilities over the course of AD. If a test is sufficiently cognitively challenging to identify individuals with MCI, it can be too difficult for individuals with moderate dementia, and *floor effects* emerge. Tests designed to characterize cognitive-communicative functioning in the later stages of dementia are generally too easy for individuals in the mild stage, and the result is a *ceiling effect*. It is the clinician's responsibility to administer measures that have demonstrated *sensitivity* for detecting the condition (MCI or AD) and high *specificity* for distinguishing it from those without the condition. Table 4–3 lists brief definitions of terms used in describing tests.

Table 4–3. Brief Definitions of Terms Related to Testing

Ceiling Effect	The failure of a test to identify the highest performance of the most competent because of a limited number of difficult test items.
Floor Effect	The failure of a test to identify the lowest possible performance because of a limited number of easy or simple test items.
Sensitivity	A statistical term that refers to the ability of a measure to correctly identify individuals who have a condition or disease.
Specificity	A statistical term that refers to the ability of a measure to correctly identify individuals who do not have a condition or disease.

Assessment of MCI Due to AD

A core clinical criterion for the diagnosis of MCI is impairment in 1 or more cognitive domains, among them episodic memory, executive function, attention, language, and visuospatial skills.[11] However, when impairment in episodic memory is present, the probability is greater that the individual has early AD. Albert and colleagues[11] have noted that individuals with MCI typically score 1 to 1.5 standard deviations (*SDs*) below age- and education-matched peers on cognitive tests. Furthermore, because the diagnosis of MCI requires evidence of "intra-individual change,"[11,p272] clinicians should schedule those who scored significantly below age- and education-matched peers for follow-up examination in 6 months or annually.

Screening for MCI

Many options are available for screening individuals for MCI. Snyder et al[15] provided a comprehensive review of 16 of 32 measures including Web-based and self-administered tools. This review was undertaken as part of the Campaign to Prevent Alzheimer's Disease by 2020 (PAD2020 initiative), in which Snyder and his team compared measures in terms of brevity, reliability, construct and predictive validity, and ease of use. Readers are referred to the PAD2020 Web site (http://pad2020.org) for details of the survey.

A non-Web-based approach to MCI screening is to use subtests from a cognitive test battery that focus on the deficits commonly observed: mental status, episodic memory, and language. After accounting for cultural or linguistic variations, individuals who fail the screening or perform in the "questionable" range should be given a comprehensive evaluation.

Mental Status Tests

Mini-Mental State Examination. The Mini-Mental State Examination (MMSE) is widely used[16,17] and evaluates orientation to person, place, and time; general knowledge; memory; communication; and copying. It requires 5 to 10 minutes to administer. The total possible score is 30, and population-based norms by age and education are available.[18] Most clinicians consider a score less than 24 as indicative of dementia[19]; however, based on results of our longitudinal studies, we suspect early dementia in literate people with scores of 25 to 26.[20] Similarly, Monsch et al[21] recommended that an MMSE score of <26 be used to indicate impairment. Of interest is a report by Tangalos et al[22] in which a decline in MMSE score of 4 or more points after intervals of 1 to 4 years was indicative of substantial cognitive deterioration. Comprehensive reviews of the psychometric properties and uses of the MMSE have been reported by Tombaugh and McIntyre[23] and Lezak et al.[24] Recently, Mitchell[25] completed a meta-analysis of 34 dementia and 5 MCI studies to determine the accuracy of the MMSE for detecting dementia and MCI and reported that the MMSE had "very limited value in making a diagnosis of MCI against healthy controls . . . and similarly limited ability to help identify cases of Alzheimer's disease against MCI."[25,p411] Mitchell concluded that the MMSE is best used to rule out a diagnosis of dementia in community and primary care settings.

Mental Status Subtest of the ABCD. The simple and reliable mental status subtest of the ABCD[1] is increasingly being used, especially by SLPs. The subtest's 13 items evaluate orientation to time, place, and person and general knowledge. It takes less than 5 minutes to give and requires no special training. The maximum possible score is 13. In the ABCD standardization study, only 5% of the normal elderly had a score below 11.5; mild AD patients averaged 9.9 and moderate AD patients averaged 4.5.

Episodic Memory Measures

Measures of Learning and Delayed Recall. A primary feature of MCI and AD is memory impairment, thus it is unsurprising that the best measures for screening for MCI and AD are tests of episodic memory.[11,26] Reports from several comprehensive longitudinal studies indicate that *initial learning of information* and *loss of information over a delay interval* are the key characteristics that discriminate between nondemented elders and those with the earliest signs of AD.[14,27–30] Examples of tests routinely used to measure a patient's ability to learn and recall information after a delay include the Logical Memory subtests (basically a story recall task) of the Wechsler Memory Scale–Revised (or other versions)[31] and the Buschke Selective Reminding Test,[32] which requires learning, storing, and retrieving information after a delay via free and cued recall and recognition. Measures similar to these can be found in the ABCD,[1] specifically the Story Retelling (Immediate and Delayed) and Word Learning subtests. Only one of these measures needs be used for screening, and the shorter test is Story Retelling (Immediate and Delayed). The ABCD will be described in greater detail in a later section of this unit, but short descriptions of the Story Retelling and Word Learning subtests follow.

Story Retelling. In this ABCD subtest, the examiner tells the patient, "I am going to tell you a short story. When I am done, I want you to tell it back to me." After the examiner reads the story aloud, the patient retells the story immediately and again after a delay of 15 minutes or more. The story contains 17 units of information. In the ABCD standardization study, normal elderly control subjects on average were able to retell 14 units of information immediately ($SD = 2.8$) and 12.4 units of information after a delay ($SD = 4.5$).

Word Learning. The ABCD Word Learning subtest involves 5 steps: controlled encoding of 16 words, a distracter task, free recall of the 16 words, use of category cues to facilitate the recall of items missed in the free-recall condition, and recognition of the 16 encoded words from among 48 words. Combining the free-recall and cued-recall scores results in a total recall score on which normal elderly control subjects achieve an average of 15. For the recognition condition, normal elderly controls score an average of 46.6 ($SD = 2.5$).

Language Measures

The literature is replete with studies in which language measures have been administered to individuals with MCI or those who have questionable AD.[33] In studies that include measures of verbal fluency, most investigators have reported finding a difference between normal elderly and those with MCI (Taler and Phillips[33] provide a comprehensive review).

Verbal Fluency. Tests of verbal fluency or generative naming are timed measures in which the subject must generate as many words as possible, beginning with a letter (usually F, A, or S) or a semantic category (eg, animals, fruits) in 60 seconds. In the Taler and Phillips[33] review of over 70 studies involving patients with MCI, a larger proportion of studies reported differences between normal controls and those with MCI using a category fluency measure than letter fluency measures. This finding was confirmed by Clark and colleagues,[34] who found greater longitudinal declines in category fluency than letter fluency in a cohort of normal elderly, preclinical AD cases, and AD patients followed for up to 5.9 years. The ABCD has a category fluency subtest.

Comprehensive Neuropsychological Approach to Screening

A definitive comprehensive cognitive test specifically designed for assessment of MCI currently does not exist. The ideal test for MCI and AD would evaluate multiple cognitive domains and allow for measurement across the clinical continuum of AD and progression into dementia. The work group on MCI,[11] rather than endorsing a single test, have cited the tests listed in Table 4–4 as valid for cognitive assessment of MCI. Until tests are designed and made available

Table 4–4. Tests/Tasks Cited by Albert et al[11] as Examples of Measures That May Be Used for Identifying Individuals with Minimal Cognitive Impairment (MCI)

Measures of Episodic Memory
Free and Cued Selective Reminding Test
Rey Auditory Verbal Learning Test
California Verbal Learning Test
Logical Memory I and II of the Wechsler Memory Scale Revised (or other version)
Visual Reproduction subtests of the Wechsler Memory Scale Revised I and II
Measures of Executive Functions
Trail Making Test
Set-shifting tasks
Reasoning tasks
Problem-solving tasks
Planning tasks
Measures of Language
Boston Naming Test
Naming tasks
Letter and category fluency tasks
Expressive speech and comprehension tasks
Measures of Visuospatial Skills
Figure copying tasks
Measures of Attentional Control
Digit Span Forward
Simple and divided attention tasks

to comprehensively assess the early subtle declines across the domains of episodic memory, executive function, language, visuospatial ability, and attention, clinicians can rely on commercially available test batteries that have been used to evaluate AD.

Montreal Cognitive Assessment

The Montreal Cognitive Assessment, version 3 (MoCA; http://www.mocatest.org),[35] was developed as a quick screening tool for mild cognitive dysfunction to assess attention and concentration, executive functions, memory, language, visuoconstruction skills, conceptual thinking, calculation, and orientation. It takes approximately 10 minutes to administer. One point is added to the sum of all subscores for an individual who has 12 or fewer years of formal education, for a total maximum score of 30 points. MoCA scores of 26 or higher are considered normal. Using the cutoff score of 26 (with 25 or below indicative of impairment), Nasreddine et al[35] found the MoCA sensitive to detecting 90% of MCI subjects, in contrast to the 18% detected by the MMSE. Rossetti et al,[36] using normative data on the MoCA collected from a large, ethnically diverse population-based sample, suggested caution in applying this cutoff score in favor of age- and education-based norms provided in their report.

Repeatable Battery for the Assessment of Neuropsychological Status

The Repeatable Battery for the Assessment of Neuropsychological Status (RBANS™)[37] was designed as a brief test to detect and characterize cognitive decline in adults ages 20 to 89 who have neurological impairment from dementia, head injury, or stroke. The RBANS has 2 parallel forms that allow for repeated evaluations to measure change in neuropsychological status over time. Five cognitive domains are evaluated: immediate memory, visuospatial/construction, language, attention, and delayed memory. Index scores corrected for age for each of the 5 domains can be derived and summed for a total score.

The RBANS has been validated for use with persons with AD.[38–41] More recently, Duff and colleagues[42] reported that individuals with MCI generally performed worse than cognitively intact peers on the RBANS and that the test was very good in terms of specificity, but its sensitivity ranged from poor to moderate. Duff et al[42] recommended that caution be used when diagnosing MCI with the RBANS. Humphreys Clark et al[43] suggested that greater diagnostic accuracy could be achieved by using percent retention scores (delayed recall score by score on final learning trial) on the Verbal Memory subtests of the RBANS in distinguishing among normal controls, individuals with MCI, and those with AD.

Assessment of AD

Screening for AD

Recall that individuals with MCI do not meet the diagnostic criteria for dementia, but many eventually go on to develop the dementia associated with AD. Therefore, the same measures used to screen for MCI are useful for screening for AD. The literature contains a number of reviews of cognitive screening instruments for use in primary care settings,[44–47] and readers are advised to seek additional information on the wide array of screening measures available by accessing these articles. Clinicians may consider the following 3 simple and quick screening measures that appear sensitive to dementia.

Memory Impairment Screen

Buschke and colleagues[48] developed the Memory Impairment Screen (MIS) as a 4-item delayed free- and cued-recall test that uses controlled learning to ensure encoding of information. The patient is presented with 4 cards, each with a word from a different semantic category. The individual is asked to read the word aloud (eg, "potato") and associate it with its semantic category cue (eg, "vegetable"). The patient is then engaged in a distracter task (counting from 1 to 20 forward and backward). Thereafter the patient is asked to freely recall the 4 items (free recall). Category cues are provided only if the item is not retrieved during the free recall (cued recall). MIS score is calculated as (2 × [free recall]) + (cued recall), resulting in scores ranging from 0 to 8. Scores of 4 or less are considered indicative of cognitive impairment sufficient to warrant comprehensive assessment. Buschke et al[48] recommend that different cutoff scores be selected depending on whether the instrument is being used for clinical or research purposes. The MIS takes approximately 4 minutes to administer and equivalent alternate forms are available.

Mini-Cog

The Mini-Cog incorporates a clock-drawing test with a simple uncued 3-item word recall task.[49] Patients are instructed to listen to and repeat 3 unrelated words, then draw a clock (which serves as the nonsemantic distracter task), and finally to recall the 3 previously presented words. The Mini-Cog takes between 2 and 4 minutes to administer.[50] Sensitivity ranges between 76% and 99% and specificity ranges between 89% and 93% depending on the characteristics of the sample being tested.[49,50] Finally, it has been shown to be valid for use in multiethnic populations.[49,51]

7-Minute Screen

Solomon and colleagues[52] selected 4 tests with previously demonstrated sensitivity to AD and ease of administration and scoring. They called the measure the 7-Minute Screen (7MS)[52] because of the time it took the average research subject to do the test. The measure consists of Enhanced Cued Recall, Category Fluency, Benton Temporal Orientation Test,[53] and Clock Drawing. Sensitivity of the screen was 92% and specificity 96% for identifying individuals with AD in a population of patients referred to a memory disorders clinic and community-dwelling control patients.[53] Recently, Ijuin and colleagues[54] reported that the sensitivity of the 7MS for detecting early-stage AD was 90.5% with specificity of 92.3%.

Comprehensive Assessment of AD

Comprehensive evaluation of cognitive-communicative functioning should provide information about the patient's mental status, verbal memory, and language-comprehension and production skills. Tests used to measure these constructs should be standardized on individuals with dementia for whom etiology and severity are specified and controlled. The ABCD[1] evaluates these constructs and was specifically designed for mild and moderate AD patients;

the Functional Linguistic Communication Inventory (FLCI)[55] evaluates language comprehension and production and was specifically designed for moderately and severely demented patients. Both are standardized batteries with demonstrated validity and reliability.

Also available are various batteries from which a clinician can fashion a test battery. The Wechsler Memory Scale–Third Edition (WMS-III)[31] is widely used to evaluate memory, as is the Rivermead Behavioral Memory Test, second edition.[56] The Block Design and Similarities subtests from the Wechsler Adult Intelligence Scale–Revised (WAIS-R)[57] have demonstrated sensitivity to early dementia and are measures of visuospatial processing and verbal associative reasoning, respectively.

As described in earlier units, individuals with AD may present with impairment in executive functioning, thus it is important to be familiar with neuropsychological tests of executive functions (Tingus et al[58] give an overview of assessment of executive function). The Wisconsin Card Sorting Test[59,60] is a widely used nonverbal test of attention and set shifting that has been administered to individuals with dementia. Other executive function tests that an SLP might administer include the Controlled Oral Word Association Test,[61] in which patients generate as many words as possible within a minute that begin with the letters F, A, and S; the Digit Span subtest of the Wechsler Adult Intelligence Scale–Third Edition (WAIS-III)[62] and WMS-III[31] in which individuals must recall number strings of increasing length; and the California Verbal Learning Test (CVLT).[63] The CVLT is a standardized memory test that assesses rate of word learning, retention after short- and long-delay intervals, semantic encoding ability, recognition memory, intrusion and perseverative errors, and response biases.

Whereas many fine aphasia test batteries exist, they were not designed for individuals with dementia. Most are too easy for mildly and moderately demented patients with AD and lack subtests of verbal episodic memory and mental status, important in differential diagnosis.

Finally, clinicians should know the Alzheimer's Disease Assessment Scale–Cognitive section (ADAS-Cog), a measure of cognitive function that has become the gold standard[64] for use in AD drug trials, as the literature is replete with references to it.[64–66] The cognitive section is one of its 2 parts and consists of measures of word recall, spoken language, language comprehension, test instruction recall, word finding, following commands, naming, figure construction, ideational praxis, orientation, and word recognition. It is scored by errors, with a maximum error score of 70. The higher the score on the ADAS-Cog, the worse the performance.

The ADAS[67, 68] combines a mental status or cognitive portion with a behavioral rating portion[69] and comprises 21 items. The entire ADAS takes approximately 45 minutes to administer and must be given by a professional trained in its administration.[69] A summary of the psychometric properties of the ADAS and ADAS-Cog has been done by Lezak et al.[24]

Arizona Battery for Communication Disorders of Dementia

The ABCD[1] consists of 14 subtests (Table 4–5) that evaluate mental status, verbal memory, and the basic skills of language comprehension and production in addition to visuospatial skill. The ABCD also contains 4 screening measures to help clinicians identify problems that can invalidate test results, including Speech Discrimination, Visual Perception and Literacy, Visual Field, and Visual Agnosia.

Standardization of the ABCD. The ABCD was standardized on individuals with AD, Parkinson's disease, and young and older nondemented community-dwelling individuals. It has also been given to individuals with multiple sclerosis[70] and Down syndrome with and without dementia.[71] The ABCD was modified for individuals in the United Kingdom,[72] Australia,[73] and the Netherlands.

ABCD subtests can be used individually or the full battery can be given. When all 14 subtests are administered, 4 types of scores are obtained: raw, summary, construct, and a total overall (Table 4–6). The full ABCD typically requires 60 to 90 minutes to complete.

Reliability of the ABCD. In the ABCD manual are data demonstrating high test-retest reliability of the battery and good internal consistency of subtests. Reliability of subtest scoring (interrater agreement) ranged from 93% to 100%.

Validity of the ABCD. Criterion validity was determined in the standardization study through correlation with 3 well-known measures of dementia severity: the Global Deterioration Scale,[74] the MMSE,[16] and the Block Design subtest of the WAIS-R.[57] Correlations among these 3 measures and ABCD subtests were high, ranging from .62 to .85.[1]

Table 4–5. The Constructs and Subtests of the Arizona Battery for Communication Disorders of Dementia (Bayles & Tomoeda, 1993[1])

CONSTRUCT 1:	LINGUISTIC COMPREHENSION
	Subtests:
	Following Commands
	Comparative Questions
	Repetition
	Reading Comprehension
CONSTRUCT 2:	LINGUISTIC EXPRESSION
	Subtests:
	Object Description
	Generative Naming
	Confrontation Naming
	Concept Definition
CONSTRUCT 3:	VERBAL MEMORY
	Subtests:
	Story Retelling–Immediate
	Story Retelling–Delayed
	Word Learning
CONSTRUCT 4:	VISUOSPATIAL SKILL
	Subtests:
	Generative Drawing
	Figure Copying
CONSTRUCT 5:	MENTAL STATUS
	Subtests:
	Mental Status

In a later, poststandardization study, Bayles et al[20] compared the ABCD with 5 measures known to be sensitive to dementia to determine which was the best for discriminating individuals with early AD from normal elders: the Block Design subtest of the WAIS-R,[57]

Table 4–6. Four Types of Scores Available from the ABCD and Their Uses

RAW	Scores on the individual subtests
SUMMARY	Standardized scores that permit performance comparisons between subtests
CONSTRUCT	Standardized scores that permit interconstruct performance comparisons
TOTAL	One score that represents performance on the entire test

the Modified Wisconsin Card Sorting Test,[75,76] a test of verbal fluency,[20] a verbal picture description test,[77] and the MMSE.[16] The ABCD was the best measure for discriminating early dementia and for distinguishing mild from moderate AD.

ABCD Subtests Most Sensitive to AD. Of the 14 ABCD subtests, Story Retelling–Delayed and Word Learning were most sensitive to AD and thus are the best for screening individuals at risk for dementing diseases. As can be seen by comparing scores in Table 4–7, the disparity in performance between normal elders and AD patients is greatest on these measures. The shorter of these subtests is Story Retelling, making it more appropriate for screening. Individuals are told a short story and asked to retell it immediately after hearing it and again after a short delay. It is quick to administer and score.

Performance of Mild AD Patients on the ABCD. The average performance of mild AD patients (mean age = 76.74 y) on ABCD subtests is charted in Table 4–7 and can be compared with the performance of normal elders (mean age = 70.44 y) and young normals (mean age = 20.29 y). Mild AD patients were significantly inferior to normal elders on all subtests except Comparative Questions, Word Reading Comprehension, and Figure Copying. However, when construct scores (composite scores) were considered, the mild AD group was, in all cases, significantly inferior in performance to normal elders. Finally, the average total overall score for individuals with mild AD was significantly lower than that for normal elders.

Performance of Moderate AD Patients on the ABCD. Moderate AD patients in the standardization study performed significantly more poorly than mild AD patients and normal elders on every ABCD subtest. Their poorest performance was on the Story Retelling task in the delayed condition.

Performance of Severe AD Patients on the ABCD. The ABCD was designed to differentiate normal elders from persons with early dementia and to track functional abilities until advanced dementia. Individuals who are severely demented find the ABCD too difficult. The FLCI[55] was developed to document their functional communication abilities.

Functional Linguistic Communication Inventory

The FLCI[55] takes approximately 30 minutes to administer and tests the following skills:

- Naming and greeting
- Answering questions
- Participating in a conversation
- Comprehending signs and matching objects to pictures
- Reading and comprehending words
- Reminiscing
- Following commands
- Pantomiming
- Gesturing
- Writing.

The FLCI score sheet enables clinicians to compare the performance of the examinee with those of AD patients in the standardization study. Also, the examinee's intact communicative functions can be charted and predictions made of skills vulnerable as AD progresses. Test results are useful in the preparation of functional maintenance programs and caregiver counseling.

The FLCI evolved from longitudinal studies of individuals with AD. It was standardized on 40 individuals with AD whose

Table 4–7. Means (*M*) for Raw, Summary, Construct, and Total Overall Scores of Young and Old Normal Control (*NC*) and Mild and Moderate (*Mod*) Alzheimer's Dementia Subjects. (Adapted from Bayles & Tomoeda, 1993.[1]) (Adapted and reprinted with Permission from PRO-ED. Copyright 1993 by PRO-ED, Inc.)

	Sign. Diff.	Young NC	Old NC	Mild AD	Mod AD
RAW SCORES	(*p* < .05)	*M*	*M*	*M*	*M*
Mental Status	2, 3	12.9	12.8	9.9	4.5
Story Retelling–Immediate	2, 3	14.9	14.0	7.3	2.6
Following Commands	1, 2, 3	9.0	8.8	8.3	6.1
Comparative Questions	3	5.9	5.9	5.7	4.6
Word Learning–Free Recall	1, 2, 3	10.4	7.6	2.3	0.8
Word Learning–Total Recall	1, 2, 3	15.7	15.1	7.7	3.3
Word Learning–Recognition	1, 2, 3	47.8	46.6	36.3	30.0
Repetition	1, 2, 3	73.7	67.9	59.2	36.8
Object Description	1, 2, 3	10.9	9.1	6.6	3.4
Reading Comp–Word	3	8.0	7.9	7.7	5.6
Reading Comp–Sentences	1, 2, 3	6.9	6.4	6.0	3.6
Generative Naming	1, 2, 3	13.4	11.4	7.1	3.1
Confrontation Naming	2, 3	18.6	18.1	15.5	8.8
Concept Definition	2, 3	57.8	56.6	41.2	10.0
Generative Drawing	1, 2, 3	13.9	12.4	10.7	5.2
Figure Copying	1, 3	11.8	11.4	11.1	6.7
Story Retelling–Delayed	1, 2, 3	14.9	12.4	1.0	0.0
SUMMARY SCORES					
Mental Status	2, 3	4.93	4.80	3.36	2.15
Story Retelling–Immediate	1, 2, 3	4.73	4.50	3.32	2.22
Following Commands	1, 2, 3	5.00	4.84	4.32	2.96

Table 4–7. (*continued*)

	Sign. Diff.	Young NC	Old NC	Mild AD	Mod AD
SUMMARY SCORES	(*p* < .05)	*M*	*M*	*M*	*M*
Comparative Questions	2, 3	4.73	4.84	4.44	3.00
Word Learning–Free Recall	1, 2, 3	4.97	4.41	2.98	2.42
Word Learning–Total Recall	1, 2, 3	4.77	4.42	2.98	2.24
Word Learning–Recognition	1, 2, 3	4.93	4.65	3.10	2.73
Repetition	1, 2, 3	4.93	4.50	3.80	2.55
Object Description	1, 2, 3	4.90	4.50	3.76	2.53
Reading Comp–Word	1, 2, 3	5.00	4.84	4.51	2.86
Reading Comp–Sentences	1, 2, 3	4.90	4.45	4.02	2.62
Generative Naming	1, 2, 3	4.83	4.42	3.54	2.27
Confrontation Naming	2, 3	4.60	4.48	3.76	2.40
Concept Definition	2, 3	4.60	4.48	3.35	1.83
Generative Drawing	1, 2, 3	4.97	4.55	4.02	2.44
Figure Copying	1, 3	4.87	4.55	4.46	2.89
Story Retelling–Delayed	1, 2, 3	4.83	4.46	3.17	3.00
CONSTRUCT SCORES					
Mental Status	2, 3	4.93	4.80	3.36	2.15
Episodic Memory	1, 2, 3	4.85	4.48	3.11	2.52
Linguistic Expression	2, 3	4.73	4.66	3.48	1.88
Linguistic Comprehension	1, 2, 3	4.91	4.69	4.22	2.84
Visuospatial Construction	1, 2, 3	4.92	4.55	4.24	2.67
TOTAL OVERALL					
Total	1, 2, 3	24.34	23.58	18.12	10.15

1 = Old NC vs Young NC	2 = Old NC vs Mild AD	3 = Mild AD vs Mod. AD

dementia severity was staged with a modified version of the Functional Assessment Stages.[78] Twenty individuals were tested twice with a 1-week interval between administrations, and high test-retest correlations were obtained for all FLCI subtests.

Patient Profiles on the ABCD and the FLCI

The test performance profiles that follow are of 3 individuals in progressive stages of AD: MCI, mild, moderate, and severe. The ABCD test scores of the individuals with mild or moderate AD will be compared with the average scores obtained by normal elders in the ABCD standardization study in 1993. The FLCI test scores of an individual with severe dementia will also be reviewed.

Mrs. G: MCI and Mild AD

Mrs. G was 80 years of age at Test Time 1. A widow for the past 10 years, Mrs. G lived independently in her home of 55 years and was still driving. She complained of memory loss that she described as difficulty retrieving names, walking into a room and not remembering what she had intended to do, and occasionally forgetting to enter purchases in her checkbook. However, she had not discussed these cognitive changes with her primary care doctor. A few months prior to her first test, Mrs. G had forgotten where she parked her car in a busy shopping mall and required the help of mall security. This concerned Mrs. G and her eldest daughter, Ann, with whom Mrs. G had almost daily contact. Ann encouraged her mother to seek a cognitive-communicative evaluation. In reviewing Mrs. G's medical history, it was noted that Mrs. G had hypertension and high cholesterol, conditions that were controlled by medication. She had had cataracts removed from both eyes at age 79 and was in good health.

Results of ABCD Testing—Test Time 1. Mrs. G was given the MMSE on the same day as the ABCD and achieved an MMSE score of 27. She was able to complete the entire ABCD in less than 75 minutes. Her raw, summary, construct, and total overall scores at Test Time 1 are presented in Table 4–8. Mrs. G's performance on the ABCD was similar to that of individuals in the older normal control group, with the exception of the Word Learning–Free Recall, Generative Naming, and Story Retelling–Delayed subtests. Although her total overall score of 21.3 on the ABCD was below the range of the older normal control group (mean [M] = 23.58; SD = 0.6), it was not in the range of mild AD (M = 18.12, SD = 2.0). This finding, along with Mrs. G's subjective complaints of memory loss, led us to recommend that she contact her physician for further medical evaluation. We also had 2 consultative sessions with Ann and Mrs. G to discuss the findings and to discuss strategies to optimize Mrs. G's functional abilities, including ways to:

- Improve comprehension by modifying language (eg, direct vs indirect; simplifying if something is misunderstood) and the communication environment (eg, limiting number of conversational partners, reducing distractions)
- Support language production by providing cues and avoidance of free-recall situations.

Mrs. G was scheduled for a follow-up evaluation in a year.

Results of ABCD Testing—Test Time 2. Ann contacted us 2 years later to request the follow-up evaluation. During the intervening time, Mrs. G had resisted Ann's efforts at medical intervention for her memory loss. Mrs. G had stopped driving at age 81 after she backed into a parked car in a grocery store parking lot. Ann was seeking confirmation of her own observations that her mother was becoming increasingly forgetful and confused. Ann also was anxious for additional strategies that would allow her mother to function and remain in her home for as long as possible.

Table 4–8 contains Mrs. G's ABCD test scores at Test Time 2. Mrs. G achieved lower raw scores on 15 of the 17 ABCD subtests, lower summary scores on 10 of 17 subtests, and lower construct scores on all 5 constructs, and her total overall ABCD score of 18.1 matched those achieved by mild AD patients (M = 18.12, SD = 2.0) in the ABCD standardization. Mrs. G's MMSE score also dropped to 24. These test results over a 2-year period documented Mrs. G's decline in cognitive-communicative abilities. The tests that continued to be the most difficult for Mrs. G were mental status and verbal episodic memory, particularly in free- and delayed-recall tasks. Her linguistic comprehension abilities remained strong.

Table 4–8. Raw, summary, construct, and total overall ABCD scores of Mrs. G at 2 test times 2 years apart shown in relation to the mean scores for elderly normal controls and mild Alzheimer's dementia subjects in the ABCD standardization.

	Elderly Normal Controls	Test Time 1 Mrs. G	Test Time 2 Mrs. G	Mild AD
RAW SCORES	M	M	M	M
Mental Status	12.8	12	10	9.9
Story Retelling–Immediate	14.0	11	8	7.3
Following Commands	8.8	9	8	8.3
Comparative Questions	5.9	6	6	5.7
Word Learning–Free Recall	7.6	5	3	2.3
Word Learning–Total Recall	15.1	14	10	7.7
Word Learning–Recognition	46.6	43	38	36.3
Repetition	67.9	67	57	59.2
Object Description	9.1	8	7	6.6
Reading Comp–Word	7.9	8	8	7.7
Reading Comp–Sentences	6.4	7	6	6.0
Generative Naming	11.4	9	5	7.1
Confrontation Naming	18.1	17	16	15.5
Concept Definition	56.6	50	43	41.2
Generative Drawing	12.4	12	19	10.7
Figure Copying	11.4	12	11	11.1
Story Retelling–Delayed	12.4	3	1	1.0
SUMMARY SCORES				
Mental Status	4.80	4	3	3.36
Story Retelling–Immediate	4.50	4	3	3.32
Following Commands	4.84	5	4	4.32

Table 4–8. (*continued*)

	Elderly Normal	Test Time 1	Test Time 2	Mild
	Controls	Mrs. G	Mrs. G	AD
SUMMARY SCORES	*M*	*M*	*M*	*M*
Comparative Questions	4.84	5	5	4.44
Word Learning–Free Recall	4.41	4	3	2.42
Word Learning–Total Recall	4.42	4	3	2.98
Word Learning–Recognition	4.65	4	3	3.10
Repetition	4.50	4	4	3.80
Object Description	4.50	4	4	3.76
Reading Comp–Word	4.84	5	5	4.51
Reading Comp–Sentences	4.45	5	4	4.02
Generative Naming	4.42	4	3	3.54
Confrontation Naming	4.48	4	4	3.76
Concept Definition	4.48	4	3	3.35
Generative Drawing	4.55	4	4	4.02
Figure Copying	4.55	5	4	4.46
Story Retelling–Delayed	4.46	4	4	3.17
CONSTRUCT SCORES				
Mental Status	4.80	4.0	3.0	3.36
Episodic Memory	4.48	4.0	3.2	3.11
Linguistic Expression	4.66	4.0	3.5	3.48
Linguistic Comprehension	4.69	4.8	4.4	4.22
Visuospatial Construction	4.55	4.5	4.0	4.24
TOTAL OVERALL				
Total	23.58	21.3	18.1	18.12

In reviewing the ABCD test results from Test Times 1 and 2 with Ann, we made several recommendations:

1. *Schedule a medical evaluation to determine whether a reversible condition was causing Mrs. G's memory decline.*
   Armed with the evaluation results, Ann set up an appointment for her mother with Mrs. G's primary care physician, who ordered a computed tomography scan of her head and blood tests. He prescribed an "Alzheimer's drug," to which Mrs. G responded well.
2. *Engage Mrs. G in activities that promote cognitive stimulation, such as an adult day care program geared for individuals with mild dementia.*
   Although Mrs. G initially resisted attending the local adult day care group, she gradually adjusted when she was given specific duties as the morning greeter and manager of the coffee cart. The adult day care program included various cognitive stimulation activities: reminiscence, choral singing, card games, coffee club to discuss current events, etc. Ann reported that Mrs. G increased her attendance in the adult day care program from 2 half days to 3 full days.
3. *Review Mrs. G's functional abilities at home and use techniques to reduce demands on impaired cognitive systems and increase reliance on spared cognitive systems.*
   We visited Mrs. G's home with Ann and discussed with her the activities of daily living that were becoming difficult. Mrs. G's ABCD results on the Word Learning–Free Recall and Word Learning–Total Recall measures at Test Time 2 showed that she was receptive to written cues, and her scores on the Reading Comprehension subtests indicated that she was able to comprehend written instructions. Ann became adept at writing clear instructions or reminders and taping them in places where Mrs. G would be sure to see them. For example, at the kitchen table, she taped a note: "Take the blue pill with your breakfast."

Mrs. J: Moderate AD

Mrs. J was 84 years old when admitted to a skilled nursing facility (SNF). She had 14 years of education and worked as an administrative secretary for 35 years. After retirement she spent time caring for her grandchildren and her husband, who passed away when she was 70. She was diagnosed with mild AD at age 79 and had been living with her eldest daughter when she suffered a fall that required hospitalization. She fell on stairs leading to the basement and whether she lost consciousness and how long she lay there were unknown. After spending 3 days in the hospital for observation, she was discharged to the SNF.

Nursing home staff referred Mrs. J for a cognitive evaluation because she seldom left her room, was socially isolated, and rarely expressed needs or communicated with other residents. The staff members inquired about ways to help Mrs. J with activities of daily living. The ABCD was administered.

Mrs. J's ABCD test results are shown in Figure 4–1. Included in the figure are her raw, summary, construct, and total overall scores. Also included are the total possible scores on each ABCD subtest and her raw score as a percentage of the total possible for each subtest. Mrs. J's total overall score of 12.4 was typical of AD patients with moderate dementia ($M = 10.15$; $SD = 3.1$) in the standardization study. Analysis of Mrs. J's ABCD test performance allowed the SLP to provide information for sections of the Minimum Data Set (MDS), the required instrument used to assess residents in Medicare or Medicaid certified nursing facilities (Table 4–9).

Mrs. J's performance on the ABCD together with results of the hearing and speech screenings were used to formulate the following long-term and short-term goals for a restorative care plan.

Long-Term Goal. Mrs. J will produce comprehensible language to express needs, participate in recognition/memory-based activities, and respond to cues to complete activities of daily living.

Short-Term Goals

1. Mrs. J will participate in twice-weekly 30-minute reminiscence groups that use recognition paradigms and faded cues to stimulate and increase verbal expression.
2. Spaced retrieval training and written cues will be used to support bathing and oral care.

Treatment Plan

Reason for Referral: Staff report that the patient rarely expresses needs or communicates with other residents, is at risk for social isolation, and requires help completing activities of daily living.

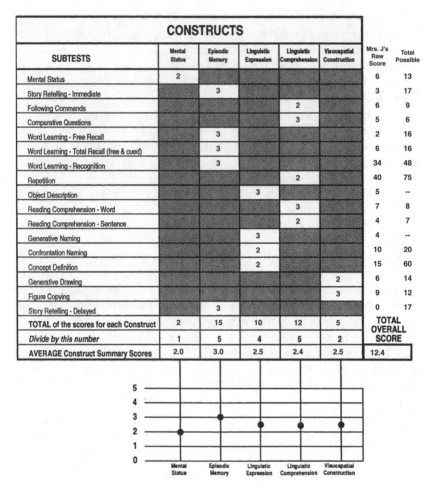

SUBTESTS	CONSTRUCTS					Mrs. J's Raw Score	Total Possible
	Mental Status	Episodic Memory	Linguistic Expression	Linguistic Comprehension	Visuospatial Construction		
Mental Status	2					6	13
Story Retelling - Immediate		3				3	17
Following Commands				2		6	9
Comparative Questions				3		5	6
Word Learning - Free Recall		3				2	16
Word Learning - Total Recall (free & cued)		3				6	16
Word Learning - Recognition		3				34	48
Repetition				2		40	75
Object Description			3			5	--
Reading Comprehension - Word				3		7	8
Reading Comprehension - Sentence				2		4	7
Generative Naming			3			4	--
Confrontation Naming			2			10	20
Concept Definition			2			15	60
Generative Drawing					2	6	14
Figure Copying					3	9	12
Story Retelling - Delayed		3				0	17
TOTAL of the scores for each Construct	2	15	10	12	5	**TOTAL OVERALL SCORE**	
Divide by this number	1	5	4	5	2		
AVERAGE Construct Summary Scores	2.0	3.0	2.5	2.4	2.5	12.4	

Figure 4–1. Mrs. J's ABCD test results shown on the ABCD Response Record Form. Note. From *Arizona Battery for Communication Disorders of Dementia (ABCD)* (p. 2), by K. A. Bayles, C. K. Tomoeda, 1993, Austin, TX: PRO-ED. Copyright 1993 by PRO-ED, Inc. Reprinted with permission.

Level of Function: The standardized ABCD was administered, which includes a speech discrimination (hearing) screen and vision screen. Patient's overall test score was similar to those of individuals with moderate dementia.

Cognition: Patient was disoriented for time and place but not for person, could recount 17% of a story immediately after hearing

Table 4–9. Relating Mrs. J's ABCD Performance to Minimum Data Set (MDS) Items

MDS Functions	Information Provided by Analyzing ABCD Performance
Ability to Recall	■ Disoriented for time and place but not for person ■ Could recount 17% of a short story immediately after hearing it; 30 minutes later, the story was entirely forgotten ■ Good recognition memory (73% accuracy) ■ Performance improves with cues
Ability to Understand Communication/Hearing Patterns	■ Can read and comprehend single words with 88% accuracy ■ Can read and comprehend sentences with 57% accuracy ■ Recognized and named items with 50% accuracy ■ Repeated with 53% accuracy ■ Able to follow 1- and 2-step commands ■ Answered comparative questions with 83% accuracy
Making Self-Understood	■ Generated 4 items in a category ■ Defined words with 25% accuracy ■ Drew simple items with 43% accuracy ■ Able to describe an object
Skills for Daily Decision Making	■ Patient was oriented for self ■ Could answer simple questions
Indicators of Disoriented Thinking	■ Disoriented for time and place

it, and remembered nothing of the story 30 minutes later. Patient demonstrated good recognition memory, and performance improved with cues.

Comprehension: Patient could read and comprehend single words and sentences with 88% and 57% accuracy, respectively, repeated with 53% accuracy, was able to follow 1- and 2-step commands, and answered simple questions with 84% accuracy.

Expression: Patient could generate 4 items in a category, defined words with 25% accuracy, drew items with 43% accuracy, and could describe 5 attributes of an object.

Speech: Normal, no dysarthria.

Hearing: Able to discriminate speech with 85% accuracy.

Overall Impression: Moderate cognitive-communicative deficit. Patient was reluctant to engage at first but became more expressive with encouragement and after achieving success with tasks less dependent on memory (eg, following commands, comparative questions).

Potential: Excellent for stated goals because of relatively intact recognition memory, ability to follow 1- and 2-step commands, good reading comprehension, and willingness to increase engagement once she has experienced success with tasks.

Severe AD: Mr. K

Mr. K was 86 years old and had been a resident of an SNF for 4 years. Mr. K had been a star baseball player in high school and college and went on to be a produce warehouse manager for 45 years. He had always been an avid gardener. For the past 2 years, Mr. K was both nonambulatory and incontinent but not bedridden. He was well liked by the SNF staff, who observed a recent change in his cognitive status. After recovering from an episode of pneumonia, Mr. K was frail and seemed less able to recognize caregivers. He had difficulty transferring from bed to wheelchair, which raised safety concerns, and his limited mobility decreased his social interactions.

Because of his cognitive status and increasing isolation, Mr. K was referred for cognitive-communicative evaluation. The ABCD was too difficult for him and he was given the FLCI. Mr. K's performance on the FLCI is shown in Figure 4–2. His total score was 35,

Performance by severity level of standardization study subjects on FLCI subtests.
Plot performance of examinee on this graph to compare examinee to AD subjects in the standardization study.

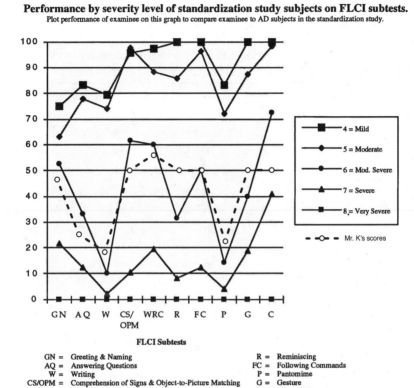

FLCI Subtests

GN =	Greeting & Naming	R =	Reminiscing
AQ =	Answering Questions	FC =	Following Commands
W =	Writing	P =	Pantomime
CS/OPM =	Comprehension of Signs & Object-to-Picture Matching	G =	Gesture
WRC =	Word Reading & Comprehension	C =	Conversation

Figure 4–2. Mr. K's FLCI test results shown in comparison to performance by severity level of standardization study subjects on FLCI subtests. Note. From *Functional Linguistic Communication Inventory (FLCI)* (p. 12), by K. A. Bayles and C. K. Tomoeda, 1994, Austin, TX: PRO-ED. Copyright 1994 by PRO-ED, Inc. Adapted with permission.

placing him in the moderately severe range. Analysis of performance allowed the SLP to provide information for sections of the MDS related to his cognitive-communicative functions (see Table 4–10).

A functional maintenance plan (FMP) was developed for Mr. K. FMPs are not carried out by the SLP but rather by support personnel and family caregivers under the supervision of the SLP. The SLP noted Mr. K's strengths and weaknesses in the FMP. His deficits

Table 4–10. Relating Mr. K's FLCI Performance to Minimum Data Set (MDS) Items

MDS Functions	Information Provided by Analyzing FLCI Performance
Ability to Recall	■ Patient has severe episodic memory problems ■ Can state and recognize written form of own name ■ Can recognize familiar objects
Ability to Understand Communication/Hearing Patterns	■ Can answer 2-choice questions with 33% accuracy ■ Can answer yes-no questions with 66% accuracy ■ Can read aloud single words with 89% accuracy ■ Can comprehend single words with 22% accuracy ■ Can name items with 22% accuracy ■ Comprehended common signs with 66% accuracy ■ Able to follow a 1-step command ■ Able to give appropriate responses during conversation about 50% of the time
Making Self Understood	■ Can write own name ■ Can pantomime the use of 2 of 9 objects ■ Can be engaged in a conversation, responded to a compliment and to the examiner's closing comment
Skills for Daily Decision Making	■ Patient was oriented for self ■ Could answer simple questions

Table 4–10. (*continued*)

MDS Functions	Information Provided by Analyzing FLCI Performance
Indicators of Disoriented Thinking	■ Disoriented for time and place
	■ Cannot respond to open-ended or multiple-choice questions, and had some difficulty with 2-choice questions
	■ Needs continuous prompting to answer questions
	■ Does not initiate conversation

were sufficiently severe that restorative therapy was not justified; nonetheless, he had retained abilities that could be used to provide quality care. He was able to:

■ Give an appropriate verbal response
■ Shake hands
■ State his name
■ Recognize written and spoken forms of his name
■ Answer some yes/no questions (2 of 3)
■ Write his name and single words to dictation
■ Recognize some signs (2 of 3)
■ Match an object to its picture (1 of 3)
■ Read single words aloud (8 of 9)
■ Comprehend some written words (2 of 9)
■ Reminisce (3 of 6)
■ Follow a simple 1-step command
■ Gesture (2 of 4)
■ Give an appropriate response to a compliment
■ Respond appropriately to a closing comment.

The SLP formulated the following long-term goal and short-term steps for maintaining Mr. K's functioning and quality of life:

Long-Term Goal. Establish routine of care that enables Mr. K to participate in daily activities that he enjoys through which he can have social interchange with caregivers and other residents.

Care Program

- Address Mr. K by name when providing care.
- Talk to Mr. K about tangible objects in the environment (eg, photograph, fruits, baseball cards, Nerf baseball) for at least 5 minutes per day and encourage Mr. K to talk about the object(s).
- Write single words on cards that relate to photos and place them where Mr. K can see them.
- Weather permitting, take Mr. K to visit the SNF's outdoor garden and allow Mr. K to tend to plants in the raised plant bed.
- Incorporate throwing and catching a Nerf baseball for at least 3 minutes each day.
- Move Mr. K to at least 3 different locations in the nursing home daily to be near people/activities and encourage him to interact with other residents and staff.
- Avoid asking Mr. K questions that demand the free recall of information.
- Use recognition and yes/no questions.
- Organize training sessions with physical therapy and care staff to train verbal cues and light touch physical cues to help Mr. K with steps for safe transfer from his bed to his wheelchair with minimal assistance.

Summary of Important Points

- Assessment of cognitive-communicative function is fundamental to the diagnosis of MCI and dementia associated with AD because cognitive decline is the defining feature of these conditions.
- It is the position of the American Speech-Language-Hearing Association (ASHA) that SLPs play a primary role in the screening, assessment, diagnosis, and treatment of cognitive-communicative disorders, including those associated with dementia.[79]
- Prior to testing an individual's cognitive communication, it is important to review the patient's medical history; check the patient's vision, hearing, and literacy; and be alert to depression and adverse drug effects on performance.
- Clinicians have options in screening for MCI. They can use subtests or specific items from a larger test battery, such as the ABCD. They can use readily available screening measures that focus on the deficits commonly observed in MCI: mental status, episodic memory, and language.

- Some commercially available test batteries have been used to evaluate AD, such as the MoCA and RBANS.
- Periodic comprehensive evaluation of cognitive-communicative functioning is an essential part of providing good patient care.
- The ABCD,[1] designed for mild and moderate patients, and the FLCI,[55] designed for severely demented patients, are standardized batteries that provide information about cognitive-communicative functioning.

References

1. Bayles KA, Tomoeda CK. *Arizona Battery for Communication Disorders of Dementia (ABCD).* Tucson, AZ: Canyonlands Publishing, Inc; 1993.
2. Cruickshanks KJ, Wiley TL, Tweed TS, et al. Prevalence of hearing loss in older adults in Beaver Dam, Wisconsin: the Epidemiology of Hearing Loss Study. *Am J Epidemiol.* 1998;148:879–886.
3. National Institute on Deafness and Other Communication Disorders. (2010) Quickstatistics. Retrieved April 5, 2013, from http://www.nidcd.nih.gov/health/statistics/Pages/quick.aspx.
4. Sharp LK, Lipsky MS. Screening for depression across the lifespan: a review of measure for use in primary care settings. *Am Fam Physician.* 2002;55:1001–1009.
5. Lamy PP. The elderly and drug interactions. *Journal of the American Geriatrics Society.* 1986;34:586–592.
6. Seymour RM, Routledge PA. Important drug-drug interactions in the elderly. *Clin Pharmacol.* 1998;12:485–494.
7. Sloan RW. Drug interactions. *Am Fam Physician.* 1983;27:229–238.
8. Larson EB, Kukull WA, Buchner D, Reifler BV. Adverse drug reactions associated with global cognitive impairment in elderly persons. *Ann Intern Med.* 1987;107:169–173.
9. Clarfield AM. The reversible dementias: do they reverse? *Ann Intern Med.* 1988;109:476–486.
10. Orange JB. Family caregivers, communication, and Alzheimer's disease. In: Hummert ML, Nussbaum, JF, eds. *Aging, Communication and Health: Linking Research and Practice for Successful Aging.* Mahwah, NJ: Lawrence Erlbaum Associates; 2001:225–248.
11. Albert MS, DeKosky ST, Dickson D, et al. The diagnosis of mild cognitive impairment due to Alzheimer's disease: recommendations from the National Institute on Aging–Alzheimer's Association workgroups on diagnostic guidelines for Alzheier's disease. *Alzh Dement.* 2011;7:270–279.

12. McKhann GM, Knopman DS, Chertkow H, et al. The diagnosis of dementia due to Alzheimer's disease: recommendations from the National Institute on Aging–Alzheimer's Association workgroups on diagnostic guidelines for Alzheimer's disease. *Alzh Dement*. 2011;7:263–269.

13. Sperling RA, Aisen PS, Beckett LA, al. Toward defining the preclinical stages of Alzheimer's disease: recommendations from the National Institute on Aging–Alzheimer's Association workgroups on diagnostic guidelines for Alzheimer's disease. *Alzh Dement*. 2011;7:280–292.

14. Locascio JJ, Growdon JH, Corkin S. Cognitive test performance in detecting, staging, and tracking Alzheimer's disease. *Arch Neurol*. 1995;52:1087–1099.

15. Snyder PJ, Jackson CE, Peterson RC, et al. Assessment of cognition in mild cognitive impairment: a comparative study. *Alzh Dement*. 2011;7:338–355.

16. Folstein M, Folstein SE, McHugh PR. "Mini-Mental State": a practical method for grading the cognitive state of patients for the clinician. *J Psychiatr Res*. 1975;12:189–198.

17. Shulman KI, Herrmann N, Brodaty H, et al. IPA survey of brief cognitive screening instruments. *Int Psychogeriatr*. 2006;18: 281–294.

18. Crum M, Anthony JC, Bassett SS, Folstein MF. Population-based norms for the Mini-Mental State Examination by age and educational level. *JAMA*. 1993;269:2386–2391.

19. Desmond DW. General approaches to neuropsychological assessment. In: Erkinjuntti T, Gauther S, eds. *Vascular Cognitive Impairment*. London, UK: Martin Dunitz; 2002:323–338.

20. Bayles KA, Tomoeda CK, Montgomery EB, Cruz, RF, Azuma T. The relation of mental status to performance on lexical-semantic tasks in Parkinson's disease. *Adv Speech Lang Pathol*. 2000;2:67–75.

21. Monsch AU, Foldi, NS, Ermini-Fünfschilling, Berres M, Taylor KI, Seifritz E, et al. Improving the diagnostic accuracy of the Mini-Mental State Examination. *Acta Neurolog Scand*. 1995; 92:145–150.

22. Tangalos EG, Smith GE, Invik RJ, et al. The Mini-Mental State Examination in general practice: clinical utility and acceptance. *Mayo Clin Proc*. 1996;71:829–837.

23. Tombaugh T, McIntyre N. The Mini-Mental State Examination: a comprehensive review. *J Am Geriatr Soc*. 1992;40:922–935.

24. Lezak MD, Howieson DB, Loring DW, Hannay HJ, Fischer JS. *Neuropsychological Assessment*. 4th ed. New York, NY: Oxford University Press; 2004.

25. Mitchell AJ. A meta-analysis of the accuracy of the Mini-Mental State Examination in the detection of dementia and mild cognitive impairment. *J Psychiatric Res*. 2009;43:411–431.

26. Rentz DM, Weintraub, S. Neuropsychological detection of early probable Alzheimer's disease. In: Scinto LFM, Daffner KR, eds. *Early Diagnosis of Alzheimer's Disease*. Totowa, NJ: Humana Press; 2000:169–189.

27. Grober E, Kawas C. Learning and retention in preclinical and early Alzheimer's disease. *Psychol Aging*. 1997;12:183–188.

28. Robinson-Whelen S, Storandt M. Immediate and delayed prose recall among normal and demented adults. *Arch Neurol*. 1992;49:32–34.

29. Rubin EH, Storandt M, Miller JP, Kinscherf DA, Grant EA, Morris JC, et al. A prospective study of cognitive function and onset of dementia in cognitively healthy elders. *Arch Neurol*. 1998;55:395–401.

30. Welsh K, Butters N, Hughes J, Mohs R, Heyman A. Detection of abnormal memory decline in mild cases of Alzheimer's disease using CERAD neuropsychological measures. *Arch Neurol*. 1991;48:278–281.

31. Wechsler D. *Wechsler Memory Scale-Third Edition*. San Antonio, TX: Harcourt Assessment; 1999.

32. Buschke H, Fuld PA. Evaluating storage, retention, and retrieval in disordered memory and learning. *Neurology*. 1974;24:1019–1025.

33. Taler V, Phillips NA. Language performance in Alzheimer's disease and mild cognitive impairment: a comparative review. *J Clin Exp Neuropsych*. 2008;30:501–556.

34. Clark LJ, Gatz M, Zheng L, Chen Y-L, McCleary C, Mack W. Longitudinal verbal fluency in normal aging, preclinical and prevalent Alzheimer's disease. *Am J Alzh Dis Other Dement*. 2009; 24:461–468.

35. Nasreddine ZS, Phillips NA, Bédirian V, et al. The Montreal Cognitive Assessment, MoCA: a brief screening tool for mild cognitive impairment. *J Am Geriatr Soc*. 2005;53:695–699.

36. Rossetti HC, Lacriz LH, Cullum CM, Weiner MF. Normative data for the Montreal Cognitive Assessment (MoCA) in a population-based sample. *Neurology*. 2011;77:1272–1275.

37. Randolph C. *Repeatable Battery for the Assessment of Neuropsychological Status*. San Antonio, TX: Psychological Corporation/ Pearson Education; 1998.
38. Freilich BM, Hyer LA. Relation of the Repeatable Battery for Assessment of Neuropsychological Status to measures of daily functioning in dementia. *Psych Rep*. 2007;101:119–129.
39. Humphreys JD, Dempsey JP, O'Bryant SE, Sutker PB. Convergent validity of the Repeatable Battery for the Assessment of Neuropsychological Status in a memory disorder clinic sample. *Arch Clin Neuropsych*. 2006;21:557–558.
40. Randolph C, Tierney MC, Mohr E, Chase TN. The Repeatable Battery for the Assessment of Neuropsychological Status (RBANS): preliminary clinical validity. *J Clin Exp Neuropsych*. 1998;20:310–319.
41. Silva ME, Humphreys JD, Dempsey JP, O'Bryant SE, Sutker PB. Test-retest reliability of the Repeatable Battery for the Assessment of Neuropsychological Status in a memory disorder clinic sample. *Arch Clin Neuropsych*. 2006;21:560–561.
42. Duff K, Humphreys Clark JD, O'Bryant SE, Mold JW, Schiffer RB, Sutker PB. Utility of the RBANS in detecting cognitive impairment associated with Alzheimer's disease: sensitivity, specificity, and positive and negative predictive powers. *Arch Clin Neuropsych*. 2008;23:603–612.
43. Humphreys Clark J, Hobson VL, O'Bryant SE. Diagnostic accuracy of percent retention scores on RBANS verbal memory subtests for the diagnosis of Alzheimer's disease and mild cognitive impairment. *Arch Clin Neuropsych*. 2010;25:318–326.
44. Ismail Z, Rajji TK, Shulman KI. Brief cognitive screening instruments: an update. *Int J Geriatr Psychiatry*. 2010;25:111–120.
45. Lorentz WJ, Scanlan JM, Borson S. Brief screening tests for dementia. *Can J Psychiatry*. 2002;47:723–733.
46. Milne A, Culverwell A, Guss R, Tuppen J, Whelton R. Screening for dementia in primary care: a review of the use, efficacy and quality of measures. *Int Psychogeriatr*. 2008;20:911–926.
47. Brodaty H, Low LF, Givson L, Burns K. What is the best dementia screening instrument for general practitioners to use? *Am J Geriatr Psychiatry*. 2006;14:391–400.
48. Buschke H, Kuslansky G, Katz M, et al. Screening for dementia with the Memory Impairment Screen. *Neurology*. 1999;52:231–238.
49. Borson S, Scanlan J, Brush M, Vitaliano P, Dokmak A. The Mini-Cog: a cognitive "vital sign" measure for dementia screening in multi-lingual elderly. *Int J Geriatr Psychiatry*. 2000;15:1021–1027.

50. Borson S, Scanlan JM, Chen P, Ganguli M. The Mini-Cog as a screen for dementia: validation in a population-based sample. *J Am Geriatr Soc.* 2003;51:1451–1454.
51. Borson S, Scanlan J, Watanabe J, Tu S-P, Lessig M. Simplifying detection of cognitive impairment: comparison of the Mini-Cog and Mini-Mental State Examination in a multiethnic sample. *J Am Geriatr Soc.* 2005;53:871–874.
52. Solomon PR, Hirschoff A, Kelly B, Relin M, Brush M, DeVeaux RD, et al. A 7-minute neurocognitive screening battery highly sensitive to Alzheimer's disease. *Archives of Neurology.* 1998;55: 349–355.
53. Benton AL. *Contributions to Neuropsychological Assessment.* New York, NY: Oxford University Press; 1983.
54. Ijuin M, Homma A, Mimura M, et al. Validation of the 7-Minute Screen for the detection of early-stage AD. *Dement Geriatr Cogn Disord.* 2008;25:248–255.
55. Bayles KA, Tomoeda CK. *Functional Linguistic Communication Inventory.* Austin, TX: Pro-Ed;1994.
56. Wilson B, Cockburn J, Baddeley A. *Rivermeade Behavioral Memory Test.* 2nd ed. Reading, UK: Thames Valley Test Co.; 1991.
57. Wechsler D. *Wechsler Adult Intelligence Scale-Revised Manual.* New York NY: Harcourt Brace & Jovanovich; 1981.
58. Tingus K, McPherson S, Cummings JL. Neuropsychological examination of executive functions. In: Erkinjuntti T, Gauthier S, eds. *Vascular Cognitive Impairment.* London, UK: Martin Dunitz; 2002:339–363.
59. Heaton RK. *Wisconsin Card Sorting Test manual.* Odessa, FL: Psychological Assessment Resources; 1981.
60. Heaton RK, Chelune GJ, Talley JL, Kay GG, Curtiss G. *Wisconsin Card Sorting Test manual:revised and expanded.* Odessa, FL: Psychological Assessment Resources; 1993.
61. Benton AL, Hamsher K deS. *Multi-lingual Aphasia Examination.* Iowa City, IA: AJA Associates; 1989.
62. Wechsler, D. *Wechsler Adult Intelligence Scale-Third Edition.* San Antonio, TX: Harcourt Assessment; 1997.
63. Delis DC, Kramer JH, Kaplan E, Ober BA. *California Verbal Learning Test®-Second Edition* (CVLT®-II). San Antonio, TX: Harcourt Assessment; 2000.
64. Sevigny JJ, Peng Y, Liu L, Lines CR. Item analysis of ADAS-Cog: effect of baseline cognitive impairment in a clinical AD trial. *Am J Alzh Dis Other Dement.* 2010;25:119–124.
65. Doraiswamy PM, Kaiser L, Beiber F, Garman RL. The Alzheimer's Disease Assessment Scale: evaluation of psychometric

properties and patterns of cognitive decline in multicenter clinical trials of mild and moderate Alzheimer's disease. *Alzh Dis Assoc Disord*. 2001;15:174–183.

66. Verhey FR, Houx P, van Lang N, et al. Cross-national comparison and validation of the Alzheimer's Disease Assessment Scale: results from the European Harmonization Project for Instruments in Dementia (EURO-HARPID). *Int J Geriatr Psychiatry*. 2004;19:41–50.
67. Rosen WG, Mohs RC, Davis KL. A new rating scale for Alzheimer's disease. *Am J Psychiatry*. 1984; 141: 1356–1364.
68. Rosen WG, Mohs RC, Davis KL. Longitudinal changes: cognitive, behavioral, and affective patterns in Alzheimer's disease. In: Poon LW, ed. *Handbook for Clinical Memory Assessment of Older Adults*. Washington, DC: American Psychological Association; 1986:294–301.
69. Weiner MF. Clinical diagnosis of cognitive dysfunction and dementing illness. In: Weiner MF, Lipton AM, eds. *The Dementias: Diagnosis, Treatment, and Research*. Washington, DC: American Psychiatric Publishing; 2003:1–48.
70. Wallace GL, Holmes S. Cognitive-linguistic assessment of individuals with multiple sclerosis. *Arch Phy Med Rehab*. 1993; 74:637–643.
71. Moss SE, Tomoeda, CK, Bayles KA. Comparison of the cognitive-linguistic profiles of Down syndrome adults with and without dementia to individuals with Alzheimer's disease. *J Med Speech Lang Pathol*. 2000;8:69–81.
72. Armstrong L, Borthwick SE, Bayles KA, Tomoeda CK. Use of the Arizona Battery for Communication Disorders of Dementia in the UK. *Eur J Dis Comm*. 1996;31:171–180.
73. Moorhouse B, Douglas J, Panaccio J, Steel G. Use of the Arizona Battery for Communication Disorders of Dementia in an Australian Context. *Asia Pac J Speech Lang Hear*. 1999;4:93–107.
74. Reisberg B, Ferris SH, de Leon MJ, Crook T. The global deterioration scale (GDS): An instrument for the assessment of primary degenerative dementia (PDD). *American Journal of Psychiatry*. 1982;139:1136–1139.
75. Hart RP, Kwentus JA, Wade JB, Taylor JR. Modified Wisconsin Card Sorting Test in elderly normal, depressed, and demented patients. *Clin Neuropsych*. 1988;2:49–52.
76. Jenkins RL, Parsons OA. Cognitive deficits in male alcoholics as measured by a modified Wisconsin Card Sorting Test. *Alc Tech Rep*. 1978;7:76–83.

77. Tomoeda CK, Bayles KA. Longitudinal effects of Alzheimer's disease on discourse production. *Alzh Dis Assoc Disord.* 1993; 7:223–236.
78. Reisberg B, Ferris SH, Franssen E. An ordinal functional assessment tool for Alzheimer's type dementia. *Hosp Comm Psychiatry.* 1985;36:593–595.
79. American Speech-Language-Hearing Association. *The roles of speech-language pathologists working with individuals with dementia-based communication disorders: position statement.* http://www.asha.org/policy; 2005.
80. Hughes CP, Berg L, Danziger WL, et al. A new clinical scale for the staging of dementia. *Br J Psychiatry.* 1982;140:566–572.
81. Mattis S. Mental status examination for organic mental syndromes in the elderly patient. In: Bellak L, Karasu TE, eds. *Geriatric Psychiatry.* New York, NY: Grune and Stratton;1976.
82. Hamilton M. A rating scale for depression. *J Neurol Neurosurg Psychiatry.* 1967;23:56–62.
83. Hamilton M. Development of a rating scale for primary depressive illness. *Br J Soc Clin Psychol.* 1970;6:278–296.
84. Beck AT, Ward CH, Mendelson M, Mock J, Erbaugh J. An inventory for measuring depression. *Arch Gen Psychiatry.* 1961; 4:561–571.
85. Zung WWK. A self-rating depression scale. *Arch Gen Psychiatry.* 1965;1:63–70.
86. Zung WWK. The Depression Status Inventory: an adjunct to the Self-Rating Depression Scale. *J Clin Psychol.* 1972;28:539–543.
87. Sunderland T, Alterman IS, Yount D, Hill JL, Tariot PN, Newhouse PA, et al. A new scale for the assessment of depressed mood in demented patients. *Am J Psychiatry.* 1988;145:955–959.
88. Alexopoulos G S, Abrams RC, Young RC, Shamoian CA. Cornell scale for depression in dementia. *Biol Psychiatry.* 1988; 23:271–284.

Unit 5

Rationale for Therapy

In the not too distant past, clinicians thought little could be done to improve the functioning of individuals diagnosed with Alzheimer's disease (AD). Early identification of those affected was not the priority it is today. However, as the number of AD patients skyrocketed, interest in early detection and intervention also skyrocketed. Worldwide, researchers in neuroscience and the behavioral and cognitive sciences focused on the disease and its management. Collectively their findings make a compelling case for early detection that can be summarized as follows:

1. The human brain is plastic, and many of the factors that advantage neuroplasticity are known.
2. Humans have multiple systems for learning and information representation that are not equally vulnerable to AD pathology.
3. Individuals with AD who have greater cognitive reserve exhibit dementia later than those with less.
4. Cognitive stimulation can improve function and produce learning (greater cognitive reserve) in individuals with minimal cognitive impairment (MCI) and AD.

Said another way, speech-language pathologists (SLPs) now have evidence-based techniques for strengthening cognitive reserve in individuals with MCI to delay conversion to dementia as well as evidence-based techniques for maximizing the functioning of those with clinically apparent AD.

Neuroplasticity

Neuroplasticity is the lifelong ability of the brain to reorganize as a result of experience.[1,2] Learning is the byproduct of neuroplasticity.

Intuitively we know this to be true because we add to and refine our knowledge throughout life. Said another way, neuroplasticity is experience dependent, and behavioral training is key to promoting brain reorganization after brain damage.[3–8]

Of significance to clinicians is the fact that the *type of experience* matters. Learning can be negative or positive. An example of negative learning is the learned non-use of a paretic limb. An example of positive learning is improvement in a language skill.

To trigger neuroplasticity, sufficient stimulation is needed, and the *type of stimulation* influences the way in which the brain reorganizes. For example, the presentation of an intensive program to incrementally challenge the auditory processing system can create structural changes in the network of cells that support auditory processing. Visual stimuli influence cell networks that support visual processing. A clinician who knows a client's profile of processing deficits and strengths can design a personalized stimulation program to influence brain response in a positive way. In the case of individuals with a neurodegenerative disease such as Alzheimer's, the goal is to strengthen residual knowledge and skills and, if possible, build additional cognitive reserve.

Table 5–1 contains a list of empirically demonstrated factors known to be influential in recovery of function.[1,9] Not listed are diet, hormones, and drugs, which also affect capacity for recovery but are not factors that SLPs manipulate.

Table 5–1. Principles of Neuroplasticity

Principle	Definition
Attention	Learning requires attention, and attention is a function of stimulus relevance to the individual.
Reward	Increases attention, and increased attention produces better learning.
Stimulation	Sensory and/or motor experience of sufficient intensity and duration are necessary for brain reorganization.
Use or Lose	Lack of use of knowledge or skills can cause their degradation.

Table 5–1. (*continued*)

Principle	Definition
Use and Improve	Use of knowledge or skills produces improvement.
Specificity	The nature of the stimulation/experience dictates the nature of brain reorganization. Example: Language stimulation produces changes in the neuronal networks that support language.
Simultaneity	Concepts, words, and actions that occur together become linked in the nervous system.
Repetition	Repetition of stimulation/experience is necessary for the creation and maintenance of long-term potentiation and learning.
Intensity	Intense experience is needed for significant brain change.
Duration	The stimulation/experience must be of sufficient duration to create lasting change.
Constrain/Forced Use	Stimulates the brain to reorganize, relearn, or compensate.
Interference	Brain reorganization in response to one experience can interfere with learning of another behavior.
Transference	Brain reorganization in response to one experience can enhance the learning of a similar behavior.
Sleep	Necessary for representation of new information and skills in the nervous system through synaptic and memory system alterations.
Age	Plasticity is greater in childhood.

Memory Systems and Their
Vulnerability to AD Pathology

In Unit 1, the various memory systems with their putative neuro-anatomical substrates were described. Of great significance to SLPs and psychologists is their differential vulnerability to the degenerative pathophysiology of AD. Whereas the neural structures supporting working and declarative memory are affected early in the disease, those supporting conditioning and motor procedural and habit memory are relatively spared.[10, 11] (For a comprehensive review of the memory deficit profile of individuals with MCI and AD, see Weintraub et al.[12])

The discovery of the differential vulnerability of the brain's representation systems to AD motivated investigations of the potential of procedural learning treatments and conditioning for improving function and quality of life for AD patients. A considerable literature now exists documenting improved skill learning in AD patients through programs that capitalized on spared procedural memory systems and conditioning.[13–19]

For individuals with MCI who have not evolved to dementia, building cognitive reserve through new learning is the primary goal. Their ability to learn new factual information will be greatly influenced by the degree of their episodic memory impairment. Early on when episodic memory is minimally affected, new fact learning will be easier. As the disease progresses, more emphasis will be placed on using spared nondeclarative memory/learning systems than on more impaired declarative systems. Regardless of stage, however, consistent use of retained skills and knowledge will help maintain them.

Cognitive Reserve

The term *cognitive reserve* refers to the mind's ability to cope with brain damage. One cannot assume that people with similar amounts of brain damage, by virtue of disease or injury, will have similar cognitive abilities. This fact is apparent in individuals with AD. Research has shown that some individuals with extensive brain pathology display few, if any, cognitive deficits in life.[20] In fact, approximately 25% of individuals with AD pathology whose brains undergo postmortem examination were symptom free in life.[21] Why the discrepancy?

Scientists theorize that some individuals may have had more neurons to begin with; others suggest that some internal or external mechanism prevents the extensive neuronal loss typical of the disease. Yet others suggest that a richer network of interneuronal connections, as a result of education and life experiences, have had a neuroprotective effect. All are true.

Katzman and colleagues[20] found an association between brain size and degree of AD symptomatology. Patients who had few symptoms and extensive pathology had higher brain weights and more neurons. More recently Perneczky[22] reported that clinical and epidemiologic studies suggest that Alzheimer's patients who have larger head sizes have better cognitive performance than those with smaller head circumferences, even though the degree of neuropathology is the same.

One "external mechanism" known to influence susceptibility to the effects of AD is amount of education. Individuals with greater education have a reduced risk for developing AD.[23-29] Further, slower decline in cognitive function has been reported in those with more education.[30-38] Similarly, people with more education and cognitively challenging careers have better cognitive reserves that reduce risk for dementia.[39-42]

Education provides cognitive stimulation, and cognitive stimulation results in synaptogenesis and a richer network of interconnected neurons, or brain reserve. Cognitive reserve is related to brain reserve (physical characteristics of brain, eg, more neurons). Brain reserve can be characterized in any number of ways, including brain size, number of neurons, synapse count, and degree of dendritic branching.

Cognitive Stimulation Therapy Can Build Cognitive Reserve

The brain needs training to maximize its potential for appropriate functional reorganization. Kleim and Jones[1] acknowledge that a better understanding is needed of when and how much training should be given for optimal response. Then, too, little is understood about how training interacts with aging, brain damage, and self-derived compensatory behaviors. Nonetheless, the fact remains that *training is needed.*

The effects of stimulation on brain reserve are easier studied in animals and indeed an extensive literature attests to their positive effects. Animals placed in rich environments have greater neuron density, dendritic branching, increased brain weight and cortical thickness than those placed in simple environments.[43-45] Hippocampal neurogenesis in the rat brain is stimulated by exercise,[46-48] learning,[49] and environmental enrichment.[50,51] These same factors produce positive results in humans though they are harder to measure. For a review of the animal literature see the paper by Jones.[45]

Treating the dementia patient poses a greater challenge than does treating an individual with a traumatic brain injury or stroke because dementia-producing diseases are usually progressive. However, as has been pointed out in earlier units, the human brain has more than one memory or learning system, and research has already shown that individuals with dementia can use these to compensate for those damaged by disease.

Another technique for providing stimulation is transcranial magnetic stimulation (TMS). Results of recent research suggest that stimulation of the brains of individuals with MCI and AD through TMS and transcranial direct current stimulation may produce significant and long-lasting beneficial changes in cognitive and motor performance. For a review of this research, see the study by Boggio et al.[52] Because these techniques are noninvasive and the results promising, more research undoubtedly will follow.

Our responsibility as clinicians is to provide stimulation that will produce positive structural and chemical changes in the brain to delay, slow, or prevent the clinical manifestation of dementia. The next unit, by Dr Kim McCullough, provides guidance about developing a cognitive stimulation program to support cognitive wellness in individuals with MCI.

Summary of Important Points

- Neuroplasticity is the lifelong ability of the brain to reorganize as a result of experience.

■ Variables shown to influence recovery of function, also known as neuroplasticity principles, include: attention, reward, stimulation, use or lose, use and improve, specificity, simultaneity, repetition, intensity, duration, constrain/forced use, interference, transference, sleep, and age.

■ Clinicians can use these principles to help clients sustain and improve their knowledge and functioning.

■ With the discovery of the differential vulnerability of the memory systems to AD pathology, clinicians can use spared systems to support and sustain the retained knowledge and skills.

■ Building cognitive reserve through new learning in individuals with MCI may delay conversion to frank dementia.

■ Sustaining function in individuals with frank dementia can improve quality of life.

References

1. Kleim JA, Jones TA. Principles of experience-dependent neural plasticity: implications for rehabilitation after brain damage. *J Speech Lang Hearing Res.* 2008;51:225–239.

2. Nudo RJ, Bury S. Motor and sensory reorganization in primates. In: Raskin S, ed, *Neuroplasticity and Rehabilitation.* New York, NY: Guilford Press; 2011:65–88.

3. Johansson, BB. Brain plasticity and stroke rehabilitation. The Willis Lecture. *Stroke.* 2000;31:223–230.

4. Johansson, BB. Guest editorial: Neurorehabilitation and brain plasticity. *J Rehab Med.* 2003;35:1.

5. Jones TA, Bury SD, Adkins-Muir DL, Luke LM, Allred RP, Sakata JT. Importance of behavioral manipulations and measures in rat models of brain damage and brain repair. *ILAR Journal.* 2003;44:144–152.

6. Jones TA, Hawrylak N, Klintsova AY, Greenough WT. Brain damage, behavior, rehabilitation, recovery, and brain plasticity. *Mental Retard Develop Dis Res Rev.* 1998;4:231–237.

7. Monfils MH, Plautz EJ, Kleim JA. In search of the motor engram: motor map plasticity as a mechanism for encoding motor experience. *Neuroscientist.* 2005;11:471–483.

8. Raskin SA, Mills GN, Garbarino JT. Practice-related changes in brain activity. In: Raskin S, ed, *Neuroplasticity and Rehabilitation.* New York, NY: Guilford Press; 2011:103–116.

9. Kolb B, Gibb R. Principles of neuroplasticity and behavior. In: Stuss D, Winocur G, Robertson I, eds, *Cognitive Neurorehabilitation*. Cambridge, UK: Cambridge University Press; 2008:6–21.

10. Salmon DP, Heindel WC, Butters N. Semantic memory, priming and skill learning in Alzheimer's disease. *Adv Psych*. 1992; 89:99–118.

11. De Vreese LP, Neri M, Fioravanti M, Belloi L, Zanetti O. Memory rehabilitation in Alzheimer's disease. *Int J Geriatr Pyschiatry*. 2001;16:794–809.

12. Weintraub S, Wicklund AH, Salmon DP. The neuropsychological profile of Alzheimer disease. *Cold Spring Harb Perspect Med*. 2012;2:a006171. doi: 10.1101/cshperspect.a006171.

13. Deweer B, Pillon B, Michon A, Dubois F. Mirror reading in Alzheimer's disease: normal skill learning and acquisition of item specific information. *J Clin Exp Neuropsych*. 1993;15:789–804.

14. Dick MB, Hsieh S, Bricker J, Dick-Muehlke C. Facilitating acquisition and transfer of a continuous motor task in healthy older adults and patients with Alzheimer's disease. *Brain Cogn*. 2003;29:294–306.

15. Dick MB, Shankel RW, Beth RE, Dick-Muehlke C, Cotman CW, Kean ML. Acquisition and long-term retention of a fine motor skill in Alzheimer's disease. *Brain Cogn*. 1996;29:294–306.

16. Deweer B, Ergis AM, Fossati P, et al. Explicit memory, procedural learning and lexical priming in Alzheimer's disease. *Cortex*. 1994;30:113–126.

17. Grober E, Ausubel R, Sliwinski M, Gordon B. Skill learning and repetition priming in Alzheimer's disease. *Neuropsychologia*. 1992;30:849–858.

18. Keane MM, Gabrieli JDE, Fennema AC, Growdon JH, Corkin S. Evidence for a dissociation between perceptual and conceptual priming in Alzheimer's disease. *Behav Neurosci*. 1991;105:326–342.

19. Verfaellie M, Keane MM, Johnson G. Preserved priming in auditory perceptual identification in Alzheimer's disease. *Neuropsychologia*. 2000;38:1581–1792.

20. Katzman R, Terry R, DeTeresa R, et al. Clinical, pathological, and neurochemical changes in dementia: a subgroup with preserved mental status and numerous neocortical plaques. *Ann Neurol*. 1988;23:138–144.

21. Ince, P. Pathological correlates of late-onset dementia in a multicenter community-based population in England and Wales. *Lancet*. 2001;357:169–175.

22. Perneczky RS, Lunetta KL, Cupples LA, et al for the MIRAGE Study Group. Group head circumference, atrophy and cognition:

implications for brain reserve in Alzheimer disease. *Neurology.* 2012;75:137–142.

23. Letenneur L, Commenges D, Dartigues JF, Barberger-Gateau P. Incidence of dementia and Alzheimer's disease in elderly community residents of south-western France. *Int J Epidemiol.* 1994; 23:1256–1261.

24. Anttila T, Helkala EL, Kivipelto M, et al. Midlife income, occupation, APOE status, and dementia: a population-based study. *Neurology.* 2002;59:887–893.

25. Zhang X, Katzman R, Salmon D, et al. The prevalence of dementia and Alzheimer's disease in Shanghai, China: impact of age, gender, and education. *Ann Neurol.* 1990;27:428–437.

26. Evans DA, Hebert LE, Beckett LA, et al. Education and other measures of socioeconomic status and risk of incident Alzheimer disease in a defined population of older persons. *Arch Neurol.* 1997;54:1399–1405.

27. Stern Y, Gurland B, Tatemichi TK, Tang MX, Wilder D, Mayeux R. Influence of education and occupation on the incidence of Alzheimer's disease. *JAMA.* 1994;271:1004–1010.

28. White L, Katzman R, Losonczy K, et al. Association of education with incidence of cognitive impairment in three established populations for epidemiologic studies of the elderly. *J Clin Epidemiol.* 1994;47:363–374.

29. Evans DA, Beckett LA, Albert MS, et al. Level of education and change in cognitive function in a community population of older persons. *Ann Epidemiol.* 1993;3:71–77.

30. Albert MS, Jones K, Savage CR, et al. Predictors of cognitive change in older persons: MacArthur Studies of Successful Aging. *Psych Aging.* 1995;10:578–589.

31. Butler, S.M., Ashford, J.W., & Snowdon, D.A. Age, education, and changes in the Mini-Mental State Exam scores of older women: findings from the Nun Study. *J Am Geriatr Soc.* 1996; 44:675–681.

32. Chodosh J, Reuben DB, Albert MS, Seeman TE. Predicting cognitive impairment in high-functioning community-dwelling older persons: MacArthur Studies of Successful Aging. *J Am Geriatr Soc.* 2002;50:1051–1060.

33. Christensen H, Korten AE, Jorm AF, et al. Education and decline in cognitive performance: compensatory but not protective. *Int J Geriatr Psychiatry.* 1997;12:323–330.

34. Colsher PL, Wallace RB. Longitudinal application of cognitive-function measures in a defined population of community-dwelling elders. *Ann Epidemiol.* 1991;1: 215–230.

35. Farmer ME, Kittner SJ, Rae DS, Bartko JJ, Regier DA. Education and change in cognitive function: the Epidemiologic Catchment Area study. *Ann Epidemiol*. 1995;5:1–7.
36. Lyketsos CG, Chen L, Anthony JC. Cognitive decline in adulthood: an 11.5-year follow-up of the Baltimore Epidemiologic Catchment Area study. *Am J Psychiatry*. 1999;156:58–65.
37. Sando SB, Melquist S, Cannon A, et al. Risk-reducing effect of education in Alzheimer's disease. *Int J Geriatr Psychiatry*. 2008; 11:1156–1162.
38. Snowdon DA, Ostwald SK, Kane RL. Education, survival and independence in elderly Catholic sisters, 1936–1988. *Am J Epidemiol*. 1989;130:999–1012.
39. Katzman R. Education and the prevalence of dementia and Alzheimer's disease. *Neurology*. 1993;43:13–20.
40. Zhang M, Katzman R, Salmon D, et al. The prevalence of dementia and Alzheimer's disease in Shanghai, China: impact of age, gender, and education. *Ann Neurol*. 2004;27:428–437.
41. Stern Y. What is cognitive reserve? Theory and research application of the reserve concept. *J Int Neuropsych Soc*. 2002;8:448–460.
42. Valenzuela MJ, Sachdev P. Brain reserve and dementia: a systematic review. *Psych Med*. 2005;35:1–14.
43. Briones TL, Suh E, Jozsa L, Woods J. Behaviorally induced synaptogenesis and dendritic growth in the hippocampal region following transient global cerebral ischemia are accompanied by improvements in spatial learning. *Exp Neurol*. 2006;198:530–538.
44. Anderson BJ, Eckburg PB, Relucio KI. Alterations in the thickness of motor cortical subregions after motor-skill learning and exercise [electronic version]. *Learn Mem*. 2002;9:1–9.
45. Jones TA. Experience-dependent changes in nonhumans. In: Raskin S, ed, *Neuroplasticity and Rehabilitation*. New York, NY: Guilford Press; 2011:103–116.
46. van Praag H, Christie BR, Sejnowski TJ, Gage FH. Running enhances neurogenesis, learning, and long-term potentiation in mice. *Proc Nat Acad Sci U S A*. 1999;96:13427–13431.
47. van Praag H, Kempermann G, Gage FH. Running increases cell proliferation and neurogenesis in the adult mouse dentate gyrus. *Nat Neurosci*. 1999;2:266–270.
48. van Praag H, Shubert T, Zhao C, Gage FH. Exercises enhances learning and hippocampal neurogenesis in aged mice. *J Neurosci*. 2005;25:8680–8685.
49. Gould E, Beylin A, Tanapat P, Reeves A, Shors TJ. Learning enhances adult neurogenesis in the hippocampal formation. *Nat Neurosci*. 1999;2:260–265.

50. Kempermann G, Kuhn HG, Gage GH. More hippocampal neurons in adult mice living in an enriched environment. *Nature.* 1997;386:493–495.
51. Komitova M, Mattsson B, Johansson BB, Eriksson PS. Enriched environment increases neural stem/progenitor cell proliferation and neurogenesis in the subventricular zone of stroke-lesioned adult rats. *Stroke.* 2005;36:1278–1282.
52. Boggio PS, Valasek CA, Campanha C, et al. Non-invasive brain stimulation to assess and modulate neuroplasticity in Alzheimer's disease. *Neuropsych Rehab.* 2011;5:703–716.

Unit 6

Cognitive Intervention and Minimal Cognitive Impairment

Kimberly C. McCullough

Evidence now exists that cognitive intervention can produce changes in the brains of individuals with minimal cognitive impairment (MCI) that are measurable through brain imaging and other biomarkers.[1,2] Intervention appears to generate the best outcomes when implemented early because individuals with MCI still retain the capability to learn and apply strategies for sustaining function. The purpose of this unit is to provide an overview of cognitive intervention programs (CIPs) and recommend key features that produce positive cognitive and/or social outcomes.

Different Forms of Cognitive Intervention Used in Individuals with MCI

Cognitive interventions have been given many names, including cognitive training, cognitive stimulation, and cognitive rehabilitation. Some focus on strengthening a particular cognitive function, such as auditory perception; others focus on strengthening an "activity," such as self-cuing. Still others are aimed almost exclusively at building a support structure for independence and well-being.[3] When developing a CIP, clinicians should rely on empirically supported training techniques and principles of cognitive intervention. Fortunately, extant data are increasing.

127

Table 6–1. Overview of Literature Regarding Cognitive Intervention Programs (CIPs)

Authors	Intensity/ Duration	Intervention	Outcome Measures	Results
Hampstead et al[13]	5 sessions within 2 weeks	Taught to use a 3-step process for object location based on a salient feature close to the object	fMRI scanning of the hippocampus in conjunction with memorizing object-location associations	Participants showed increased activity within the left hippocampal body for both the trained and untrained stimuli
Barnes et al[10]	100 minutes per day, 5 days per week for 6 weeks	Intensive, computer-based cognitive training designed to improve processing speed and accuracy through several tasks that changed difficulty	Repeatable Battery for Assessment of Neuropsychological Status (RBANS, main measure), California Verbal Learning Test–II (CVLT-II), Controlled Oral Word Association Test (COWAT), Boston Naming Test (BNT), Delis-Kaplan Executive Function Scale (California Trail Making and Fluency tests), Spatial Span Test	Participants showed significant improvements in verbal learning and memory

Study	Training schedule	Intervention	Outcome measures	Results
Belleville et al[8]	One 2-hour session weekly for 8 weeks	Teaching episodic memory strategies, metacognition, and computer-based training of attention	Three tasks of episodic memory (list recall [Côte-des-Neiges Computerized Memory Battery], face–name association, and text memory), Questionnaire d'Auto-évaluation de la Mémoire, computerized adaptation of the Brown-Peterson technique	Participants showed significant improvements in delayed list recall and face–name association. Improved subjective memory and well-being also noted.
Kinsella et al[17]	5 weekly 1.5-hour sessions	Education about memory, external memory aids, and general coping strategies	Tests of Prospective Memory Performance (Reminding Task from the Rivermead Behavioural Memory Test, envelope task), Multifactorial Memory Questionnaire (Ability, Strategy, and Contentment subscales), Strategy Knowledge Repertoire	Participants showed significant improvements in actual performance of everyday memory as indexed by prospective memory tasks.

Systematic literature reviews provide data summaries of the most effective training techniques and principles used in CIPs.[4-7] Stott and Spector[4] reviewed 10 studies designed to reduce memory impairment and/or develop compensatory strategies in individuals with MCI and reported that the most successful interventions were those that were individually tailored to the person. Investigators used both objective and subjective measures, and all reported positive responses on the subjective measures.[4] In many studies, benefits were also apparent on objective measures of processing speed, attention, and episodic and working memory.[5] The greatest improvements were seen on measures of language abilities. Surprisingly, however, protocols with longer sessions and/or duration of training did not necessarily achieve larger effect sizes.

Improvements in brain imaging and biomarker detection technology techniques have vastly improved our understanding of the neurological responses to cognitive intervention and how such responses can have neuroprotective effects. Nonetheless, data to date are insufficient to answer the following questions:

1. What types of training are best for various deficit profiles?
2. What outcome measures are most sensitive and valid?
3. Is individual treatment better than group or a combination approach?
4. How long should stimulation sessions last?
5. How long should the program last?
6. How long will program effects, when present, last?

That these questions remain unanswered is understandable because of the variability across studies in the number of cognitive processes addressed, the criteria for measuring progress, intensity and duration of treatment, and mode of treatment delivery (individual or group). But whereas differences in methods, measures, and outcomes have left many important questions unanswered, a very positive message is difficult to overlook. All meta-analyses and reviews report improvements from CIPs and highlight their potential to delay or prevent cognitive decline and functional disability in persons with MCI (Table 6–1 presents an overview). Furthermore, key elements have emerged that can assist clinicians in designing, evaluating, and implementing intervention.

1. Use a repetition-based intervention that targets specific (identified during assessment) cognitive domains with an emphasis on sensory processing (eg, auditory and visual).
2. Provide direct training of strategies and functional skills (eg, memory strategy training and decision making).
3. Empower clients with education regarding healthy aging and brain habits.
4. Include opportunities for social engagement.

Belleville and colleagues[8] investigated the efficacy of a CIP for individuals with MCI that included components from each of these key elements. Their program comprised the training of attention (2 sessions), the teaching of different episodic memory strategies (5 sessions), and the provision of education regarding memory and aging (1 session). The intervention was administered across 8 weekly sessions that lasted approximately 120 minutes. Training was conducted in groups of 4 to 5 participants. Each key element was isolated and addressed during individual sessions and not intermixed with other session elements. Despite the short amount of exposure, results indicated significant effects on 2 outcome measures: delayed list recall and face–name association. Moreover, a significant effect was observed on subjective measures of memory and well-being, indicating that the group setting had a positive impact overall on these participants.

Karow et al[9] used a similar treatment protocol that also contained each of the aforementioned key elements. In contrast to Belleville et al's CIP,[8] the speech pathologists included key elements within each session. The intervention was administered across 10 weekly sessions that lasted approximately 120 minutes. Training was conducted in groups of 5 to 7 participants. Performance gains were noted on objective and subjective measures. The MCI participants showed the most improvement in the areas of language and executive functions. Thus, various approaches can be used and appear to be productive if the key elements are included.

Key Element 1: Base repetition focus on cognitive domains.

Implementation of a repetition-based intervention that targets specific cognitive abilities with an emphasis on sensory processing (eg, auditory, visual) is crucial to building cognitive reserve in individuals with MCI. Furthermore, results of studies suggest that more practice leads to more resilient learning. These sessions are similar to the typical "work-out" session at a gym. However, rather than targeting muscle groups, the focus is on repeated practice of specific cognitive abilities. The targeted cognitive domains can be stimulated through traditional methods, such as paper-pencil tasks and face-to-face drill, or through computer-based training. Regardless of the method used, the treatment should be tailored to the patient's pattern of impairments to strengthen functions that are still relatively well preserved.

Computer-Based Training

Many clinicians use computer-based cognitive training programs because they are cost-effective, provide multiple training options, and are easily accessed in the clinic and at home. Computer programs provide instant feedback to both the client and the speech-language pathologist, allowing for immediate, objective review of performance data. Nonetheless, the expertise of the speech-language pathologist is needed to select appropriate goals for the needs of the individual, evaluate progress, and make program modifications that advantage continuous progress.

Barnes and her colleagues[10] investigated the efficacy and feasibility of using an intensive computer-based home training program to improve processing speed and accuracy in auditory processing. All program participants were provided an at-home computer and access to Posit Science Corporation software. MCI participants used the program for 100 minutes per day, 5 days per week for 8 weeks. The software used by the intervention group was designed to target processing speed and auditory working memory. The control group was given computer-based assignments that included listening to audio books, reading online newspapers, and playing visuospatially oriented computer games. The control group participated for 90 minutes per day, 5 days per week for 8 weeks. The researchers used the Repeatable Battery for the Assessment of Neuropsychological Status (RBANS) as the primary outcome measure of global cognitive functioning. Although no statistically significant difference in scores on the RBANS was found between the intervention and control group, the authors did note some interesting patterns of improvement. Effect size for measures of verbal and visual working memory consistently improved in the intervention group. In contrast, effect size for measures of language and visuospatial function showed improvement trends in the control group. Overall, results from this study highlight the concept of neuroplasticity, that the brain is malleable and continuously changing and the type of input received determines the nature of change. These results also draw attention to the importance of including treatment activities and stimuli relevant to the client. In this study, the control group essentially had the same treatment schedule, but the content included more opportunities for selecting topics of interest. Clinicians should work diligently to ensure that treatment is individualized to their clients.

Rosen and colleagues[11] conducted a similar study with 6 individuals with MCI using the same cognitive training software program. Of interest was whether the effects of stimulation would be detectable through functional magnetic resonance imaging (fMRI) measurements. They were. The authors reported enhanced left-anterior hippocampal activation as well as a performance improvement on the RBANS. This study provides further evidence that individuals with MCI retain sufficient neuroplasticity to benefit from cognitive stimulation training.

Li and colleagues[5] recommend computer-based interventions for improving specific cognitive domains and confirm that improvements can be documented with objective clinical measures. However, when focusing on direct strategy training and social engagement, clinicians should also use subjective measures of performance. Thus, even if one is able to improve cognition with computer training and verify the improvement through objective measures, individuals with MCI may not clearly see the benefit unless the intervention is meaningful to their everyday lives. The clinician is well advised, therefore, to provide a multidimensional approach that enables clients to share their perspectives on the value of the training program.

Key Element 2: Provide direct training of strategies and functional skills.

Particularly troubling to many individuals with MCI is prospective memory (remembering to remember). Consequently, providing direct training of strategies to enhance prospective memory is useful for everyday memory competence.

Nearly half of the studies reviewed by Jean and colleagues,[6] in their review of cognitive intervention programs for MCI, emphasized training mnemonic strategies. Statistically significant improvements were often reported on objective measures of memory after training. Furthermore, results of many studies indicate that memory strategy training positively impacted other cognitive domains. Additionally, MCI participants reported statistically significant improvements on subjective measures of memory and quality of life after cognitive interventions that included memory training.

Other investigators[12] have used fMRI to provide empirical support for direct training of strategies as a treatment for individuals with MCI. Small group sessions (4 to 5 people) of 2 hours duration were held weekly for 6 weeks. Sessions focused on mnemonics and techniques to promote elaborate encoding and retrieval. During the first session, participants learned about memory and aging. The following 5 sessions promoted episodic memory training through the use of interactive imagery, method of loci, face–name associations, hierarchical organization, and semantic organization techniques. In participants with MCI, comparison of positive clinical outcomes with fMRI results revealed significant changes in a large brain network that included regions typically associated with memory. Based on these results, the authors concluded that increased brain activation occurred in areas related to the taught intervention. Importantly, the memory training normalized the brain activation deficits associated with MCI. Thus, after intervention, the brain activation levels in the MCI group were similar to those of the control group. This finding provides further evidence that the MCI brain remains plastic and can change (and improve) with intervention.

Hampstead and colleagues[1,13] conducted a randomized, single-blind study to evaluate the value of a mnemonic strategy for encoding and retrieving the location of objects. Participants with MCI and healthy older controls were randomly assigned to a mnemonic strategy training or exposure group. The researchers created a computerized "virtual" home with 9 rooms. The mnemonic strategy intervention consisted of a series of steps in which participants identified a salient feature in each room that was close to the target object and then verbally linked the object to the room. Thereafter, they were instructed to create a detailed mental image (or "movie") of the object, room feature, and fact linking the object to the room. Participants in the repeated exposure group were given an opportunity to learn the location of each object. Thereafter, they were shown each object and asked to identify its location. In both the MCI participants and healthy older controls, results indicated that mnemonic strategy training was superior to exposure, with benefits that were still measurable at least 1 month after training. Before training, fMRI scans of MCI participants revealed reduced hippocampal activity during encoding and retrieval. Following mnemonic strategy training, the MCI group had increased hippocampal activity during encoding and retrieval, as well as improved delayed memory scores, as measured by the RBANS. Increased hippocampal activation was not observed in subjects in the MCI group who received exposure but not the mnemonic strategy training.

Key Element 3: Empower clients with education regarding healthy aging and brain habits.

Lifestyle factors such as physical activity, healthy diet, and stress reduction are important to healthy aging, and many cognitive stimulation programs include an education component. Individuals with MCI can benefit from adopting healthy habits that reduce their risk for dementia. Examples of topics addressed include: (1) health benefits of physical activity and ways of integrating physical activity into the individual's lifestyle; (2) stress and depression, their causes and management; and (3) the benefits of sleep and management of sleep disturbances. Interested family can be included in the education sessions, as can other professionals—for example, dietitians, physical therapists, and exercise physiologists, who can become a long-term resource to affected individuals.

Key Element 4: Include opportunities for social engagement.

An early sign of cognitive impairment is a decrease in level of activity and withdrawal from social activities. These changes can be so subtle that family members and even the individuals with MCI may be unaware of them. Kaye and colleagues[14] studied the activity levels and degree of participation in social activities of 28 individuals with MCI and reported a decline in time spent out of the home compared with cognitively intact participants.

To stimulate social engagement, many investigators have used a group format in their cognitive intervention program, among them Kurz and colleagues,[15] who provided a 4-week, 4-hour-a-day group program to individuals with MCI and those with mild dementia. Participants planned leisure activities and discussed methods for strengthening their social network. They received group training on stress reduction and management, relaxing, improving their memory, exercise, and the use of external memory aids. After 4 weeks, the MCI participants showed significant improvements on measures of activities of daily living, mood, and verbal and nonverbal episodic memory. In contrast, participants with mild dementia exhibited a nonsignificant increase in verbal memory but no other changes.

Rapp and colleagues[16] conducted a randomized clinical trial to evaluate a multicomponent CIP that comprised 6 weekly sessions lasting 2 hours each and included group training about memory, relaxation skills, and mnemonic strategies. At the conclusion of training, participants' subjective perception of their memory capacities was improved, although no improvement was apparent in memory performance. However, in the follow-up memory probe, there was a trend toward better word list recall in the delayed condition by MCI participants compared with controls. Results of these studies demonstrate the viability of a group format for providing education and cognitive stimulation.

Conclusion

The growing awareness by the public of the value of cognitive stimulation to build cognitive reserve will increase the demand for cognitive training programs. SLPs can be involved in planning and overseeing these programs, especially if they advocate for early identification of MCI and engage in screening of late-middle-aged and older individuals who are hospitalized, or residents of assisted living facilities, those who come to the clinic for hearing tests, or who accompany spouses with communication disorders to the clinic.

Summary of Important Points

- Intervention appears to generate the best of outcomes when implemented early because individuals with MCI still retain the capability to learn and apply strategies for sustaining function.

- When developing a cognitive intervention program, clinicians should rely on empirically supported principles and training techniques of cognitive intervention.
- Key elements have emerged to assist clinicians in designing and implementing intervention.
  - Use a repetition-based intervention that targets specific (identified during assessment) cognitive domains with an emphasis on sensory processing (eg, auditory, visual).
  - Provide direct training of strategies and functional skills (eg, memory strategy training and decision making).
  - Empower clients with education regarding healthy aging and brain habits.
  - Include opportunities for social engagement.

References

1. Hampstead BM, Stringer AY, Stilla RF, et al. Activation and effective connectivity changes following explicit-memory training for face-name pairs in patients with mild cognitive impairments: a pilot study. *Neurorehab Neural Repair*. 2011;210–222.
2. Belleville S, Bherer L. Biomarkers of cognitive training effects in aging. *Curr Transl Geriatr Gerontol Rep*. 2012;104–110.
3. Clare L, Woods RT. Cognitive training and cognitive rehabilitation for people with early-stage Alzheimer's disease: a review. *Neuropsych Rehab*. 2004;14:385–401.
4. Stott J, Spector A. A review of the effectiveness of memory interventions in mild cognitive impairment (MCI). *Int Psychogeriatr*. 2011;23:526–538.
5. Li H, Li J, Li N, Li B, Wang P, Zhou T. Cognitive intervention for persons with mild cognitive impairment: a meta-analysis. *Ageing Res Rev*. 2011;10:285–296.
6. Jean L, Bergeron M-È, Thivierge S, Simard M. Cognitive intervention programs for individuals with mild cognitive impairment: systematic review of the literature. *Am J Geriatr Psychiatry*. 2010;18:281–296.
7. Simon SS, Yokomizo JE, Bottino CMC. Cognitive intervention in amnestic mild cognitive impairment: a systematic review. *Neurosci Biobehav Rev*. 2012;36:1163–1178.
8. Belleville S, Gilbert B, Fontaine F, Gagnon L, Ménard E, Gauthier S. Improvement of episodic memory in persons with mild cognitive impairment and healthy older adults: evidence from a

cognitive intervention program. *Dement Geriatr Cogn Disord.* 2006;22:486–499.

9. Karow CM, Harvey J, Helm-Estabrooks N, Bloom C, Cuellar M. *Cognitive Decline in Normal Aging and Mild Cognitive Impairment.* Presented at conference of the American Speech-Language-Hearing Association, San Diego, CA, 2011.

10. Barnes DE, Yaffe K, Belfor N, et al. Computer-based cognitive training for mild cognitive impairment: results from a pilot randomized, controlled trial. *Alzh Dis Assoc Disord.* 2009;23:205–210. doi: 10.1097/WAD.0b013e31819c6137

11. Rosen AC, Sugiura L, Kramer JH, Whitfield-Gabrieli S, Gabrieli JD. Cognitive training changes hippocampal function in mild cognitive impairment: a pilot study. *J Alzh Dis.* 2011;26:349–357.

12. Belleville S, Clément F, Mellah S, Gilbert B, Fontaine F, Gauthier S. Training-related brain plasticity in subjects at risk of developing Alzheimer's disease. *Brain.* 2011;134:1623–1634.

13. Hampstead BM, Stringer AY, Stilla RF, Giddens M, Sathian K. Mnemonic strategy training partially restores hippocampal activity in patients with mild cognitive impairment. *Hippocampus.* 2012;22:1652–1658.

14. Kaye JA, Maxwell SA, Mattek N, et al. Intelligent systems for assessing aging changes: home-based, unobtrusive, and continuous assessment of aging. *J Gerontol.* 2011;66B(suppl 1):80–90.

15. Kurz A, Pohl C, Ramsenthaler M, Sorg C. Cognitive rehabilitation in patients with mild cognitive impairment. *Int J Geriatr Psychiatry.* 2009;24:163–168.

16. Rapp S, Brenes G, Marsh AP. Memory enhancement training for older adults with mild cognitive impairment: a preliminary study. *Aging Ment Health.* 2002;6:5–11.

17. Kinsella GJ, Mullaly E, Ong B, et al. Early intervention for mild cognitive impairment: a randomized controlled trial. *J Neurol Neurosurg Psychiatry.* 2009;80:730–736.

Unit 7

Treatment: Direct Interventions

*D*irect interventions are those in which clinicians provide individual or group therapy to individuals with AD to enable them to maintain residual knowledge and skills. *Indirect* interventions are modifications of the physical and/or linguistic environments to support cognition and communication.

Federal legislation in the form of the Omnibus Budget Reconciliation Act of 1987,[1] which governs accreditation of long-term care facilities, requires that residents be comprehensively evaluated and care plans developed that will enable them to function at their highest level of ability. Today, speech-language pathologists (SLPs) routinely receive reimbursement for assessing patients' ability to improve. If improvement is expected and the special skills of the SLP are needed, claims reviewers will approve "restorative therapy" and the clinician will be reimbursed.[2] When a patient's restoration potential is judged insufficient after a trial of restorative therapy, the clinician can develop a functional maintenance plan (FMP). The time involved in plan development and the time needed to instruct supportive personnel in carrying it out plus periodic oversight are reimbursable services if the FMP is created during the period of diagnostic or restorative therapy.

Definitions

Restorative therapy—Therapy in which clients are brought to the functional level they are capable of but have not been achieving.

Functional maintenance plan (FMP)—An FMP is a plan of care designed to maintain clients at a particular level of functioning.

Treatment Guidelines

Regardless of the cause of dementia, clinicians will find the following guidelines helpful in designing a care plan for maximizing function:

1. Strengthen the knowledge and processes that have the potential to improve.
2. Reduce demands on impaired cognitive systems.
3. Increase reliance on spared cognitive systems.
4. Provide stimuli that evoke positive fact memory, action, and emotion.

Identifying the profile of preserved knowledge and skills is as important to therapy planning as identifying deficits because spared systems can be used to compensate for those impaired. As previously noted in Unit 3, the memory deficit profile of individuals with AD changes over the disease course. The primary problem of early-stage patients is impaired episodic memory, thus demands on it need to be reduced throughout the disease course. Other declarative memory systems (semantic and lexical) are relatively functional in the early and middle stages of the disease but gradually deteriorate. Working memory is compromised, however, but environmental supports can help maintain orientation and focus attention. Best preserved throughout the disease are nondeclarative memory systems (conditioning, procedural learning, priming), and they can be used to teach new behaviors[3]; see De Vreese et al[4] for a review.

Care should be taken when planning therapy to use stimuli that evoke positive emotion and action. Neither individuals with dementia nor their caregivers benefit from the creation of a negative emotion in the patient. Negative moods often persist long after the provoking stimulus is forgotten, increasing caregiver stress and staff time and diminishing the quality of life of the patient.

Strategies for Successful Intervention

In addition to using the principles of neuroplasticity to guide therapy planning, 3 other factors need consideration: perceptibility of stimuli, span capacity of working memory, and task complexity.

Facilitating Perception

Aging significantly affects human sensory systems and perception. Diminished perception impedes learning because perception is the first step in information processing. An awareness of how aging affects sensory systems is needed to help elders compensate. The sensory systems most influential in information processing are the visual and auditory systems.

Vision and Aging

According to the 2010 National Health Interview Survey, 12.2% of the noninstitutionalized American population 65 to 74 years of age and 16.1% of individuals 75 and over report vision loss or trouble seeing even when wearing glasses or contact lenses. The best-known age-related change in vision is loss of focusing power, a condition known as *presbyopia*.[5] Although the eye stops growing in adolescence, the lens continues to grow in adulthood, becoming denser and less elastic. The result is that elders are less able to focus and need 2 to 3 times more light than a person 20 years of age.[6] Aging also affects the ability to adjust to changes in levels of illumination. In youth, one can go from a sunny afternoon to a darkened movie theatre and quickly accommodate the change in illumination. With age, this adjustment is slower and less efficient, leaving individuals temporarily blind. Finally, age-related changes in vision affect the ability to perceive patterns and increase the need for contrast to aid perception.[7]

Many elders develop age-related cataracts, glaucoma, macular degeneration, and diabetic retinopathy.[8,9] With cataracts, vision becomes blurred. People who have cataracts say it is like looking at the world through a cloud or thick haze. Glaucoma also causes blurred vision and loss of peripheral perception. Macular degeneration is the condition in which degeneration occurs in the center of the retina. The result is a blind spot in the center of the visual field. Macular degeneration is also associated with increased sensitivity to light and altered color vision.[10]

Individuals with Alzheimer's disease (AD) experience these age-related changes in vision plus others that are disease related, specifically, deficits in color discrimination and contrast sensitivity.[11,12] Of clinical significance is how sensory loss can negatively affect the ability to communicate, perform tests, and carry out daily activities. Consider that vision is needed to read lips, recognize facial expressions, interpret contexts, follow directions, and read. People with impaired depth perception, a decreased ability to focus, and reduced sensitivity to contrast may appear more demented than they really are because sensory losses diminish performance on tests and activities of daily living (ADLs). Even young adults who wear glasses often remark that they have trouble hearing and thinking without their glasses. Unfortunately, the need for accommodations that will enhance vision is underappreciated by many professional and personal caregivers. In short, impaired vision reduces patients' quality of life, increases their dependency, and makes them appear more intellectually impaired than they are by virtue of neuropathology.

Managing Problems with Vision to Facilitate Learning. First and foremost, clinicians need to screen for vision problems. A simple screening technique is included in the Arizona Battery of Communication Disorders of Dementia (ABCD).[13] However, clinicians without access to the ABCD can easily create a similar one. Type a variety of letters on a page of paper turned horizontally. Repeat one letter, like *A*, several times in each quadrant of the page. Have the examinee identify all the *A*'s in each quadrant. Note whether the target letter is unnoticed in an area of the page. Also note whether the individual has to move the paper to find the *A*'s. If so, a visual field defect may be present, and the patient should be referred for neurologic evaluation.

Before neuropsychological testing, ensure that patients who need glasses wear them. Use printed materials that are in large font size and colors that provide strong contrast (black on white or vice versa) to make print perceptible. Because of the frequency of vision problems, clinicians should introduce themselves when greeting a client. Although elders may be able to see them, they may be unable to discern their facial features sufficiently to recognize them. Finally, do not stand in front of a window or bright light when talking to an elder, as glare can reduce perception of your face. It is important for individuals with dementia to have adequate light throughout the day. "Sunlight starvation" negatively impacts the health and quality of life of many elders.[6,14]

Lack of sunlight disturbs circadian rhythms that regulate a host of biological processes,[7,15] among them body temperature, hormone release, heart rate, blood pressure, and the sleep–wake cycle. Sunlight also benefits the body's immune system. In addition to the negative effects of sunlight deprivation on bioregulatory processes, victims of sunlight starvation are at greater risk for depression and sleep disorders that can diminish cognitive functioning. Increased agitation is also a by-product of light deprivation,[16] and investigators have demonstrated that exposure to bright light can reduce agitation and improve sleep–wake cycles even in late-stage dementia patients.[17,18]

Brawley[7,p87] recommended the following guide for lighting in long-term care facilities. Her recommendations are of value to SLPs and other personnel responsible for the care of elders:

- Raise the level of illumination.
- Provide consistent, even light levels.
- Eliminate glare.
- Provide access to natural daylight.
- Provide gradual changes in light levels in transition spaces.
- Provide focused task lighting.
- Improve color rendition from lamps or light sources so that colors of the environment and people in the environment are not distorted.

Color and Vision. Not only does the lens of the eye thicken with age, it yellows, filtering out the short wavelengths. The consequence is distortion of color perception, particularly after age 60.[19,20] Discriminating along the blue–yellow axis is particularly affected, as is discriminating among light colors. AD patients are less able to distinguish between blue and green hues and between blue and violet hues. Most resistant to age effects are the ability to discriminate the red hue and the brightness of color.[21] By providing high contrast, clinicians can increase function (Figures 7–1 and 7–2). For example, table tops and countertops should contrast strongly with the color of the floor. Dishes that contrast with the color of the table facilitate eating. The best contrast is provided by using a dark color against a light background or vice versa (eg, black against white, light yellow against dark blue). Poor contrasts result from dark green against bright red, yellow against white, blue against green, and lavender against pink.

Hearing and Aging

Hearing loss is the most prevalent disability of elderly Americans.[22–24] According to the National Health Interview Survey,[25] presbycusis, or age-related hearing loss, affects approximately 18%

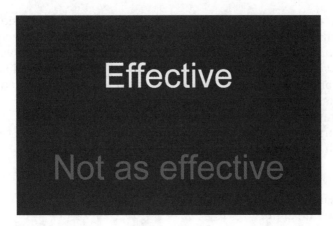

Figure 7–1. Example of high and low letter contrasts.

of individuals in the United States age 65 years or older. Cruick-shanks et al[26] conducted a population-based study of 4541 people age 48 to 92 and reported the prevalence of all degrees of hearing loss to be 45.9% among those 65 years and older. Among nursing home residents, the percentage appears to be even higher, approaching 90%.[27] In addition, adults with hearing loss often experience further deterioration of hearing ability with advancing age.[28]

Hearing loss in persons with AD is not less prevalent than in nondemented elders,[29] and some researchers suggest that it may be more prevalent.[29,30] Indeed, Uhlmann et al[31] found that the risk for dementia increased with progressively greater amounts of hearing loss. It has been reported that between 70% and 80% of nursing home residents have hearing loss.[32–34] Gold et al[35] documented the prevalence of hearing loss in 94% of a sample of individuals with AD. Just as a deficit in vision can make individuals with dementia seem more intellectually and functionally impaired than they are, so also can a deficit in hearing.[31,34,36,37] Yet, it is shocking how few investigators have controlled for the hearing abilities of individuals with dementia in neuropsychological and treatment studies. Additionally, without correction, hearing loss can contribute to more rapid cognitive decline. Using longitudinal data from individuals with AD, Uhlmann et al[38] observed that cognitive decline over a

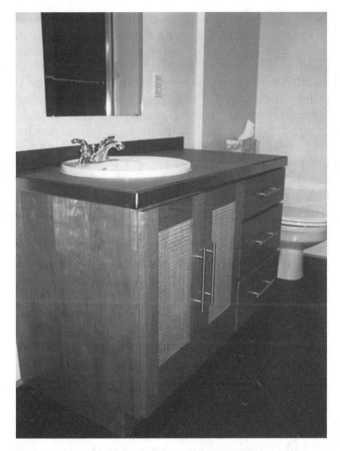

Figure 7–2. Example of bathroom with high contrast between sink and countertop and between toilet and floor.

1-year period was almost twice as great in the group of hearing-impaired people with AD than in the nonhearing-impaired AD group.

Furthermore, when individuals with dementia receive amplification, their cognitive and behavioral functioning improves.[34,38–41] Palmer and colleagues[42] documented reduction in problem behaviors reported by caregivers for all 8 AD subjects in their study after hearing aid use. Allen and associates[39] reported improvement on measures of hearing handicap over 24 months of hearing aid use in their study of 31 individuals with dementia.

Before making a judgment about the existence and severity of dementia in any individual, hearing should be tested. If comprehensive assessment of hearing is possible, clinicians may wish to follow the procedures described by Mahendra et al,[43] in which otoscopy, pure-tone threshold testing, word recognition testing, and the Hearing Handicap Inventory for the Elderly–Screening Version[44] were used. If comprehensive hearing assessment is unavailable, clinicians can screen hearing by simply administering a speech discrimination test (repeating spoken words or judging whether 2 spoken words are the same) in the environment in which the testing will occur. Regardless of dementia severity, most individuals with AD can complete a simple speech discrimination test.[13]

To facilitate hearing, clinicians should:

- Have clients who need hearing aids wear them
- Eliminate noise
- Ensure that clients can see their face
- Amplify their voice.

Consider Span Capacity of Working Memory

Working memory span capacity, or the ability to hold incoming information in consciousness, attenuates slightly with age and markedly in individuals with dementia.[45,46] Reduction in span capacity can affect an individual's ability to comprehend task instructions. Daneman and Carpenter[47] documented that a large span capacity for auditory-verbal information is associated with better language comprehension than a small span capacity. Having knowledge of a patient's span capacity for verbal and visual information is important in designing tasks that will not be so overwhelming that they discourage participation. Often, when dementia patients are given more information than they can process, they withdraw.

Span capacity for verbal and visual information can be tested with the Digit Span and Spatial Span subtests of the Wechsler Memory Scale–Third Edition.[48] The Digit Span subtest involves having patients repeat strings of numbers that increase in length (forward) and in reverse order (backward). In the Spatial Span subtest, span capacity for visual information is tested by having patients touch a sequence of blocks of increasing length in the same order as presented by the examiner and in reverse order.

Control of Task Complexity

Match task demands to the ability of the client. Consider the number and type of mental operations required to complete the task and the level of complexity of the stimuli. Recall tasks, in which learners have to search memory for answers, are widely recognized as more difficult than recognition tasks.[49-51] Because of their serious episodic memory deficit, tasks that rely on recent memory will position the AD patient to fail.

Bayles et al[52] conducted a research study that enabled them to compare the difficulty of a variety of communication tasks. They administered 11 different tasks all of which use the same 13 conceptual stimuli to AD patients in the order shown in Table 7–1. Stimulus equivalence across tasks enabled them to make intertask comparisons of difficulty. The most difficult tasks were superordinate and coordinate naming that required recall of conceptual information. In superordinate naming, study subjects had to grasp the relation between the stimulus concept and the larger category of things to which the stimulus concept belonged, retrieve the superordinate, and express it orally. This task placed demands on working memory span, attention, and decision making, as well as on

Table 7–1. Tasks and Concepts Used in the Bayles Study[52]

Confrontation Naming	Pencil
Auditory Comprehension	Comb
Dictation	Hanger
Oral Reading	Mask
Definition	Racquet
Reading Comprehension	Dart
Coordinate Naming	Harmonica
Superordinate Naming	Domino
Superordinate Identification	Knocker
Pantomime Expression	Stethoscope
Pantomime Recognition	Compass
	Tongs
	Abacus

lexical and semantic memory. In coordinate naming, study subjects had to grasp the relation between the stimulus concept and other objects in the same category and provide the names of coordinates. Like superordinate naming, this task taxed working and semantic memory systems.

Least difficult of the tasks were oral reading of words, auditory comprehension, and reading comprehension, the latter 2 being multiple-choice tasks that required recognition of the answer rather than recall. Oral reading is a mechanical task that does not require comprehension of the words or manipulation of information.

Concept difficulty also affected performance. Less common concepts were those most likely to elicit an error. The concepts of compass, stethoscope, and abacus accounted for most errors, and "pencil" and "comb" elicited the fewest errors. In sum, remember:

- Recognition is easier than recall.
- Comparing features of items is harder than item recognition.
- Expressing relationships is harder than confirming relationships.
- The more cognitive manipulations needed to do the task, the harder the task.
- Complexity of stimuli interacts with task complexity.
- Visibility of instructions enhances performance.

Minimize Error Responses

Dementia patients with episodic memory deficits typically forget their error responses. Consequently, they do not self-correct as neurologically normal adults do in trial and error learning.[53] When an error response is repeatedly given, its engram is strengthened, making it more accessible in the future. In recent years a substantial body of evidence has demonstrated that errorless learning (EL) procedures can be used to teach a variety of tasks to individuals with memory problems.[54] EL procedures are those that provide sufficient cuing or scaffolding to minimize errors, with gradual fading of cues as the target is learned. Guessing is discouraged. Whereas trial and error learning requires self-insight and monitoring, EL is less effortful. Clare and Jones[55] note its usefulness for individuals with diminished executive functions and poor error monitoring.

To reduce the probability of error response, the clinician can manipulate stimulus characteristics and response contingencies. The technique of vanishing cues has frequently been used to reduce the production of errors in amnesic individuals.[53,55–58]

In the vanishing cues technique, learners are given strong cues at first. Gradually, cue strength is reduced until the target response is given in the absence of cues. For example, if you wanted to teach the patient that the name of the night nurse was Janet, you could present the name in its full form on a card and ask the patient to read the card to answer the question "What is the name of your night nurse?" On subsequent learning trials, the patient would read a card with the name in a reduced form (Jane, Jan _ , Ja _ _ ,). The vanishing cues method has been used successfully in demented[59,60] and nondemented amnesic patients.[61-63]

Recognition Is Easier Than Recall

Free recall of information is harder than recognizing information. All students know the truth of this statement. A multiple-choice test is easier than an essay test because it contains the correct answers that have only to be recognized. Answering an essay question requires an effortful search of memory and formulation and generation of a coherent, correct response.

Like students, dementia patients perform better on recognition tests. Table 7–2 shows the performance of mild and moderate Alzheimer's patients and young and older normal individuals on tests of free recall, cued recall, and recognition. As the data show, the

Table 7–2. Mean raw scores and standard deviations (*SD*) of young and old normal control subjects and individuals with mild and moderate Alzheimer's disease (*AD*) on the Word Learning Subtest of the ABCD. Cued recall is Total Recall–Free Recal.

	Young Normal M(SD)	Old Normal M(SD)	Mild AD M(SD)	Moderate AD M(SD)
Word Learning– Free Recall	10.4(2.1)	7.6(2.5)	2.3(1.9)	0.8(1.2)
Word Learning– Total Recall	15.7(0.6)	15.1(1.2)	7.7(3.9)	3.3(3.6)
Word Learning– Recognition	47.8(0.6)	46.6(2.5)	36.3(7.7)	30.0(7.1)

ability to freely recall information diminishes with age. The performances of healthy adults and those with dementia were better in the cued recall and recognition conditions. Note that to determine the effect of cued recall, subtract the free recall score from the total recall score.

A simple technique for preserving the dignity of individuals with AD who have severe episodic memory problems is to avoid questions like, "What's new?" or "What have you been doing?" or "What did you have for dinner?" These require the recall of recent events. Recognition questions that require yes/no answers are much easier—for example, asking, "Did you go to the store today?" "Is that a new dress?" or "Does dinner with the Smith's sound like fun?" Choice questions such as, "Would you like fish or chicken for dinner?" "Shall we watch television or go for a walk?" have the answer in the questions, making them easier.[64]

Use Retrieval Cues That Reflect Support Given at Encoding

The amount of informational overlap between a retrieval cue and the memory engram established at the time of encoding is vital to memory proficiency. This is known as the *encoding specificity principle*.[65] A substantial literature exists demonstrating that recall is improved when retrieval cues reflect support given at encoding.[66–68] All of us are familiar with detectives having witnesses return to the scene of a crime as a memory trigger. Many of us have experienced the same phenomenon at high school and college reunions. Back at our alma maters, surrounded by old friends, we recall events we likely never would have thought of again had we not returned to the setting in which they occurred. Most of us are familiar with the phenomenon of being at a loss for how to answer a test question if the question is worded differently from how the information was presented in class. Therefore, to facilitate recall, use retrieval cues that reflect support given at the time of encoding.

Allow More Time to Respond

Information processing slows with age. Birren et al[69] demonstrated that between the ages of 65 and 91, slowing of psychomotor speed occurs even in healthy elders and adversely affects performance on neuropsychological tests. However, when healthy elders are given sufficient time to respond, they often perform like young adults, and the age effect disappears. Dementia patients are slower in processing as a function of age and as a function of pathology that has disrupted their neurochemistry and interfered with intercellular communication. To reduce task complexity, allow more time for responding.

Avoid Having Client Multitask

As we know from personal experience, tasks requiring division of attention or alternating attention are harder. Because of their deficits in attention and memory, dementia patients have much greater difficulty with dividing their attention than healthy adults.[70,71] Researchers have demonstrated that the neural activation associated with a given task decreases in healthy adults if a second task is done at the same time.[72-74] The same is true for individuals with dementia. Filoteo and colleagues[75] reported that individuals with AD were better at focusing attention on a single aspect of a stimulus than dividing attention between 2 aspects of the same stimulus. Camicioli et al[76] observed that AD patients slowed their walking speed when asked to perform a verbal fluency task (reciting male names) while walking.

The popular activity of texting or being on the computer while doing something else is multitasking and requires dividing one's attention. Research has shown that the "timesaving" technique of multitasking makes healthy adults less efficient[77,78] and consumes more time. In fact, the process of switching back and forth between tasks can take longer than doing one task to completion and then doing the next task because the brain has to overcome "inhibitions" imposed to stop the first task to do the second task. Newman and colleagues[77] had subjects listen to sentences while comparing rotating objects. When done together, the resources available for processing visual input dropped 29%. Brain activation for listening dropped 53%. Ophir et al[78] found that media multitaskers were more susceptible to interference from irrelevant environmental stimuli and irrelevant representations in memory and they performed worse on task switching. In sum, multitasking can cause attention gaps, stress, trouble concentrating, and problems with recent memory. To reduce task difficulty for the dementia patient, avoid multitasking.

Using the Principles of Neuroplasticity to Support Learning and the Maintenance of Knowledge and Skills

Attention

The first step in providing a direct intervention is to secure the client's attention. Attention is a function of the relevance of the stimulus or activity to the individual and whether it is associated with reward. Perlmuter and Monty[79] observed that personalizing a task through patient choice increased engagement, motivation, and performance. Interview clients and caregivers about activities enjoyed premorbidly and goals they want to achieve. Then, by being offered a choice of activities, patients gain a sense of control over their learning. Similarly, familiarity with the premorbid interests of the client enables clinicians to provide desired rewards.

Reward and Emotion Are Related

Emotion affects perception, guides attention, and ultimately modulates behavior.[80] Individuals are continuously in a state of allocating their finite attentional resources to particular stimuli, and they do so according to how incoming stimuli are prioritized.[81] Stimuli that are pleasurable, unique, and/or threatening attract our attention. Emotional memory enables us to recognize danger.[82-84] Thus events, people, and objects with emotional significance are more memorable and produce changes in brain chemistry that facilitate learning.[85-88] LaBar et al[89] demonstrated that emotionally charged information captures the attention of dementia patients better than neutral information. In their study, individuals with AD and normal controls were shown pairs of visual scenes, some emotionally charged, some neutral. Recordings of eye movements revealed that AD patients, like normal controls, were more attentive to the emotionally charged scenes. Moayeri et al[90] presented AD subjects with stories accompanied by slides containing either emotionally charged or neutral elements. Although AD patients were inferior to normal controls at recalling both types of story elements, emotional passages were better remembered than neutral ones.

Music Stirs Emotion and Enhances Memory

Emotional memories are easier to recall than unemotional[85–87] and music elicits emotion.[86,91–93] These facts formed the basis of a study of the effect of music listening on autobiographical recall and the number of emotional words used in the recounting of auto-biographical memories in individuals with AD and healthy older adults.[86] Haj et al[86] reported that autobiographic recall was significantly improved after listening to music, especially music chosen by the subjects compared with Vivaldi's *Four Seasons* and silence. Significantly more memories were recalled after listening to music than after silence and significantly more were remembered after listening to chosen music than the *Four Seasons*. Also, more emotional words were produced by individuals with AD than healthy elderly, especially in the chosen condition.

Stimulation

The purpose of direct intervention is to stimulate the use of retained knowledge and skills and learn compensations for those lost. Among the stimulation techniques that are supported by evidence are 3 that are useful for individuals with cognitive deficits: priming, active engagement, and elaborate encoding.

Priming

The phenomenon of advantaging a response, by virtue of prior exposure to the target or a related item, is called *priming*. Priming is demonstrated empirically by an increase in the frequency, speed, or accuracy of a response as a consequence of prior exposure to a particular stimulus.[94,95] Recent exposure to a word, concept, or proposition makes the word, concept, or proposition more likely to come to mind. For example, if you have recently seen the word "desert," you will recognize it more quickly on tasks requiring you to make judgments about it (eg, whether it is a real word). You will also make faster judgments about the words "hot" and "dry" because they are associated with the concept of desert. The prior exposure to the word "desert" heightened the level of activation of the concept 'desert' and its lexical representation. It also heightened the level of activation of related concepts and their lexical representations. The heightened activation of "desert," "hot," and "dry" occurred without your awareness and is the result of the spreading activation of energy within semantic and lexical memory.

Storms[96] conducted one of the early studies that fueled interest in the phenomenon of priming. Students were asked to study a list of words (List A), all of which elicit high-frequency associations. For example, the word "eagle" typically elicits the word "bird." Then Storms presented the students with a second list of words (List B), which were high-frequency responses to the words on List A but do not usually elicit words on the A list. For example, the List A word "eagle" elicits "bird," but the word "bird" (List B) does not usually elicit the word "eagle." However, Storms observed that the production of words on List A, as responses to the words on the List B, was significantly higher when List A had been previously seen. Cofer[97] subsequently labeled this phenomenon as "priming of associations." Over the decades, the term *priming* has been extended to refer to a variety of events, or paradigms, that facilitate the production of target information.

Repetition or Direct Priming

Repetition, or direct priming, refers to the paradigm in which an item presented in the training (or study phase) of an experiment is identical to or composed of fragments of the target item to be produced. For example, exposure to the word "boat" in the training phase will result in faster judgments about the word "boat" when it is seen again. Or prior exposure to the word "boat" will result in individuals saying "boat" when later shown the fragment "bo_ _ ." Repetition, or direct priming, is perceptual; that is, it is modality specific and independent of the meaning of the item. Commonly used repetition priming tasks require subjects to complete a word, make a decision about a word, or identify previously seen words.

Associative or Indirect Priming

Associative, or indirect, priming refers to the paradigm in which the item presented in the training phase is associated with the item to be produced. Associative/indirect priming is conceptual or semantic. Commonly used indirect, associative priming tasks are word associations, category production, and general knowledge tests. In word association tasks, a word presented in the training phase produces a preference for an associated word. For example, the word "snow" produces a preference for "cold."

In category production tasks, the subject is presented with items from a particular category—for example, fruits—and later asked to generate as many exemplars of fruit as possible. The prior exposure to items from the category increases the likelihood that they will be produced later in the category production task.

In a general knowledge task, the prior presentation of a word increases the probability of it being given as the answer to questions related to the word. For example, prior exposure to the word "saguaro" will increase the probability that saguaro will be given as an answer to the question, "What is a large cactus that grows in southern Arizona?"

Using Priming Clinically

Many SLPs are unfamiliar with the term *priming* but routinely use priming to facilitate the performance of clients through cuing. Clinicians often give an associate of a word to facilitate its recall ("use it to cut through wood" for "saw"). Often, they provide the name of the larger category of things the target word belongs to ("it's a form of transportation" for "car"). Sometimes they provide the opposite of a word to stimulate the target ("up" for "down").

Clinicians use more than words to prime desired behavior, among them routines, memory books, music, and contexts. A routine is a behavioral chain in which each behavior functions as a discriminative stimulus for the next behavior and a conditioned reinforcer for the previous link.[98] Ylvisaker and Feeney[99] described routines as concrete structured event complexes that become organized mental representations that cue behavior.

Wallets and memory books with photographs of past events and loved ones, together with text, have been demonstrated to improve the meaningfulness of verbiage produced by dementia patients in conversation.[100-102] The photographs and text in the memory wallets and books activate memories and prime associations with the pictured events and people.

All of us have memories and emotions associated with music. Thus, music used as a prime can transport us to a past event. If the event is positive, our mood may improve. Music is a tool clinicians can use because evidence shows that musical memory is better preserved than other types of semantic memory.[103] The ability to remember melodies and lyrics is retained even in some severely demented individuals. Some investigators argue that musical semantic memory appears to be an "island" of cognitive preservation.[104,105] Foster and Valentine[92] used music to facilitate autobiographic recall in individuals with dementia. They observed increased arousal and interest when background music was played during recall. Mahendra[106,107] also used music to stimulate the recall of autobiographical events in individuals with dementia and observed greater animation, increased verbal output, and greater physical action (imitating drum playing, toe tapping, and in one case, dancing). As noted, Haj et al[86] reported that music stimulated autobiographical memory and that music chosen by the patient was better than the opus *Four Seasons*.

Context can also cue behavior. Recognition of this fact has led clinicians to train individuals in the contexts in which the desired behavior is needed. This is important because skills acquired in a clinical context often do not transfer to real-world contexts.[108]

Active Engagement

For healthy individuals and dementia patients, learning is both faster and better when the individual is actively engaged in the learning process.[68,109] Active engagement in its fullest form is learning by doing. Action-oriented learning involves the nondeclarative procedural memory system that enables us to develop skills and habits. This system is generally preserved in individuals with AD.[110,111] If individuals are provided the opportunity to practice new procedures, such as making transfers from a wheelchair, they become habitual and increase independence. Further, by providing opportunities for the execution of previously learned procedures, this knowledge can be sustained.[112,113]

Self-Generation of a Response

One technique for actively involving dementia patients is to have them generate a response during learning rather than just watching and listening. This "generation effect" was first described by Slamecka and Graf,[114] who observed that young adults had better memory for words they generated, in response to cues, than for words they simply heard. Mitchell et al[115] reported the same effect in old and young adults and individuals with AD. Study participants read 30 sentences in subject-verb-object (SVO) form and generated the object in another 30 SVO sentences (eg, "The gentleman opened the _____."). Later they were presented with the verbs from the 60 sentences and asked to supply the objects associated with them. Study results showed that individuals with AD, like healthy young and older adults, better remembered self-generated objects than those already present in the stimulus sentences they read.

Lipinska et al[116] conducted a study in which they provided a 20-page booklet to individuals with AD. On each page was the name of a concrete noun. Patients had to generate "general properties" of 10 of the nouns. For the other 10, they had to make yes/no judgments about whether the item was a member of the category provided by the experimenter. At recall, the AD patients were provided the properties they generated for 10 of the words, and experimenter provided cues for the remainder. Recall was best when subjects responded to their self-generated properties. Opportunities to use retained knowledge can be provided through reminiscence sessions, cooking, and community activities.

More recently, researchers demonstrated that active involvement during the study phase of a word-stem completion task significantly improved performance.[117] The word-stem completion priming rates of AD patients in a variety of encoding conditions were compared. When they had to make semantic judgments about the words or generate words in the encoding phase, they performed virtually equivalent to healthy elders; however, when they only read or rated the words, word-stem completion priming was inferior to that of healthy elders.

Reminiscence

Reminiscence therapy stimulates recall.[118] When individuals with dementia and healthy adults are presented with pictures, newspaper articles, video clips, clothes, and props associated with a theme, their personal experiences related to the theme come to mind.[119] Sheridan[120] recommends using a variety of materials to trigger all the senses. A synergy can develop in reminiscence sessions in which group members aid each other in the recall of past events. When one member of the group shares a memory, it stimulates memories in other group members.

Good reminiscence sessions require planning.[121] In addition to selecting a theme and obtaining related tangibles, the clinician should develop a list of questions that probe for the obvious and less obvious recollections individuals are likely to have. Plan how to include all group participants. For example, have some individuals describe a tangible item and then ask other members what they think about the tangible. Group members can share the responsibility for reading newspaper articles or article headlines. Finally, reminiscence can be a stimulus for physical activity such as dancing, food preparation,[122] or exercise.

Good Themes for Reminiscence Sessions

- Culturally appropriate holidays
- Personal milestone events (getting married, graduation)
- Notable world events
- Weather events
- National traditions
- Geography

Elaborate Encoding

Elaborate encoding, or greater depth of processing of information, builds stronger engrams for the information. Healthy elders show improved memory when strategies such as visual imagery and organization of information to be learned are provided during encoding.[123–125] Such strategies promote a greater depth of processing; and the greater the depth of processing of the to-be-retained information, the greater the learning. Good teachers know the truth of this principle.

The depth-of-processing principle also applies to individuals with AD (see the study by Bäckman and Small[126] for a review). Bird and Luszcz[127] observed that AD patients learned better when they were engaged in tasks like thinking of attributes of the to-be-remembered target or its category membership compared with trying to recall pictures in the absence of any type of cue. Similarly, Herlitz and Viitanen[67] noted improved learning when material to be remembered had a logical structure. Arkin et al[128] found that working within a semantic schema by linking a target to its superordinate category facilitated learning.

Glasgow et al[129] developed a technique, known as the PQRST method (Preview, Question, Read, State, Test), for increasing the depth of information processing. The PQRST method is a systematic way of involving the learner actively in encoding. First, the information is previewed. Next, the learner is asked to answer questions about it. Thereafter, the learner reads the information, summarizes it, and is subsequently tested. A similar technique is having learners listen to text, identify key propositions, and later use them in a story they create.[130]

Another technique for learning text is to divide it into segments and have the learner summarize each before proceeding to the next segment. Stevens et al[131] used question asking and reading (QAR) to increase memory for the content of stories. The reading of the text was distributed among group members and scripted to include text-based questions that group members had to answer. The QAR technique increased the learning of text and the frequency of verbal interactions among group members.

A three-step strategy for making face-name associations was described by McCarthy.[132] First the learner identifies a prominent facial feature, then transforms the name into a concrete image, and finally formulates an interactive visual image of the two elements (feature and image of name).

Repetition

When individuals repeatedly access information and bring it to conscious awareness, the engram for the information is strengthened, making it more accessible for future recall.[133] All of us learned the importance of this fact as students. The more frequently we thought about the information presented in lectures and class exercises, the more likely we were to recall it on a test. Just as repetition helps healthy individuals learn information and skills, it also helps memory-impaired individuals learn.[134] Many researchers have demonstrated that repetition facilitates learning in dementia patients.[107,135–137] If the information to be learned is new, as opposed to previously known information, learning will be slower and forgotten more quickly. For some dementia patients, new fact learning is impossible. When this is the case, the clinical focus will be on maintaining preserved knowledge (eg, names of grandchildren, how to make a 911 call) through repeated opportunities to use it.

Spaced Retrieval Training (SRT)

Spaced retrieval training (SRT) is a repetition-based shaping procedure in which an individual is asked to recall information (eg, a name, procedure, location) over increasingly longer intervals of time.[138] It is a simple procedure requiring little cognitive effort from the patient.[139] SRT can be nested in other activities such as conversation, physical therapy, or doing a craft project and used by both personal and professional caregivers.[138]

Clinicians control the type of target response, duration of the intervals between retention probes, and the number of learning trials. The first intervals between recall probes are very short and gradually extended. When an incorrect response is given, the clinician returns to the length of interval that last produced a correct response. Activities during the intervals between retention probes can be related to the desired response or unrelated.

Originally described by Landauer and Bjork in 1978,[140] SRT was not used with a dementia patient until 1985. Since then, its efficacy has been explored by many investigators, who report success in teaching face–name associations,[141–144] object location,[142] object names,[141,146–148] and various verbal and motor responses.[147–150] Brush and Camp[151] used SRT to teach 7 dementia patients and 2 memory-impaired stroke patients 3 pieces of information: the therapist's name, a fact important to the person (eg, room number, spouse's birthday), and a compensatory technique for improving communication. Five participants with dementia completed the study and all learned the 3 pieces of information, as did the 2 stroke patients. However, participants had varying levels of recall a month later. Davis et al[152] tested the efficacy of using spaced retrieval to teach previously known but forgotten personal information in a randomized placebo-controlled study of 37 AD patients. Cognitive stimulation served as the placebo and consisted of home-administered attention exercises. AD patients in the intervention group improved in the recall of personal information during the 5-week intervention, whereas the performance of patients in the placebo group remained constant.

The efficacy of spaced retrieval with dementia patients is thought to result from spared nondeclarative memory processes that enable individuals to learn associations even though they cannot remember the event of learning.[153] A common question is, How long does a dementia patient remember what is learned through SRT? Researchers have reported retention of information for many months in some individuals with dementia. In these cases, the individuals had frequent occasions to use the learned information. If the information to be learned is not needed, and therefore never accessed, it will not be retained long.

Examples of Uses for SRT

Both fact knowledge and procedures can be taught with SRT. Examples of useful facts are: previously known but forgotten personal information; name–face associations of caregivers and family members; location of important objects; 911 as an emergency number. Examples of useful procedures are: making a phone call for help; making a safe transfer; finding an important location (eg, bathroom, bedroom, nurses' station, dining room); increasing volume of voice; operating a faucet; and inserting a hearing aid.

Intensity, Duration, Constraint

To date, studies have not been done on the effects of therapy intensity and duration on the communicative functioning of individuals with AD. However, the behavioral responses of the client and performance on outcome measures provide evidence as to the adequacy of intensity and therapy duration. When a client loses interest in a session or shows signs of fatigue, intensity should be lowered or the session terminated. Duration of restorative therapy is largely dependent on whether the client makes demonstrable progress. Common sense suggests that a single weekly session is unlikely to result in significant progress. Daily sessions that provide distributed practice are more likely to produce measurable results.

Summary of Important Points

- Direct interventions are those in which clinicians provide individual or group therapy to individuals with AD to enable them to maintain retained knowledge and skills.

■ Federal legislation requires that residents of long-term care facilities have a care plan that will enable them to function at their highest level of ability.
■ SLPs routinely receive reimbursement for providing direct interventions that improve the communicative functioning of individuals with dementia.
■ Four guidelines are helpful in designing a care plan for maximizing patient function:
   ■ Strengthen the knowledge and processes that have the potential to improve.
   ■ Reduce demands on impaired cognitive systems.
   ■ Increase reliance on spared cognitive systems.
   ■ Provide stimuli that evoke positive fact memory, action, and emotion.
■ To improve learning, take the following into account when planning intervention:
   ■ Facilitate perception.
   ■ Control task complexity.
   ■ Work within memory span.
   ■ Minimize error responses.
   ■ Recognition of information is easier than free recall of information.
   ■ Use retrieval cues that reflect support given at encoding.
   ■ Allow more time to respond.
   ■ Avoid having client multitask.
   ■ Use multimodal stimulation.
   ■ Make therapy personally relevant.
■ To support learning and the maintenance of skills, incorporate some of the following principles of neuroplasticity when planning intervention:
   ■ Attention.
   ■ Use emotion to capture attention.
   ■ Provide cognitive stimulation.
   ■ Priming facilitates recall.
   ■ Actively engage the patient in learning.
   ■ Reminiscence.
   ■ Provide opportunity for elaborate encoding to build strong engrams.
   ■ Provide opportunity for repetition of information to be learned or strengthened.
   ■ Consider the effects of therapy intensity and duration.

- The human brain continuously remodels its neural circuitry as a function of experience. Neural circuits not actively engaged will ultimately degrade.
- With greater understanding and awareness of this fact, the demand for cognitive stimulation to facilitate the remodeling of neural circuitry will dramatically increase.

References

1. Omnibus Budget Reconciliation Act of 1987. Public Law No. 100–203, 483.15; 1987.
2. American Speech-Language-Hearing Association. *ASHA's Medicare Handbook for Speech-Language Pathologists*. Rockville, MD: Author; 2004.
3. Salmon DP, Heindel WC, Butters N. Semantic memory, priming and skill learning in Alzheimer's disease. *Adv Psychol*. 1992; 89:99–118.
4. De Vreese LP, Neri M, Fioravanti M, Belloi L, Zanetti O. Memory rehabilitation in Alzheimer's disease. *Int J Geriatr Psychiatry*. 2001;16:794–809.
5. National Center for Health Statistics. *National Health Interview Survey*. Retrieved 2011 from http://www.cdc.gov/nchs/nihs.htm.
6. Clark L. *The Ancient Art of Color Therapy*. New York, NY: Pocket Books; 1975.
7. Brawley E. *Designing for Alzheimer's disease*. New York, NY: John Wiley & Sons; 1997.
8. Prevent Blindness America. *Vision Problems in the U.S.: Prevalence of Adult Vision Impairment and Age-Related Eye Disease in America*. 4th ed. Schaumburg, IL: Author; 2008.
9. Schieber F. Vision and aging. In: Birren JE, Schaie KW, eds, *Handbook of the Psychology of Aging*. 6th ed. Burlington, MA: Elsevier; 2006:129–161.
10. Fangmeier R. *The World Through Their Eyes: Understanding Vision Loss*. New York, NY: The Lighthouse; 1994.
11. Cronin-Golomb A, Corkin S, Growdon JH. Visual dysfunction in Alzheimer's disease: relation to normal aging. *Ann Neurol*. 1991;29:41–52.
12. Cronin-Golomb A, Sugiura R, Corkin S, Growdon JH. Incomplete achromatopsia in Alzheimer's disease. *Neurobiol Aging*. 1993;14:471–477.

13. Bayles KA, Tomoeda CK. *Arizona Battery for Communication Disorders in Dementia.* Austin, TX: Pro-Ed; 1993.
14. Campbell SS, Kripke DF, Gillin JC, Hrubovcak JC. Exposure to light in healthy elderly subjects and Alzheimer's patients. *Physiol Behav.* 1988;42:141–144.
15. Salgado-Delgado R, Osorio AT, Saderi N, Escobar C. Disruption of circadian rhythms: a crucial factor in the etiology of depression. *Depr Res Treatm.* 2011;2011:1–9.
16. Satlin A, Volicer L, Ross V, Herz L, Campbell S. Bright light treatment of behavioral and sleep disturbances in patients with Alzheimer's disease. *Am J Psychiatry.* 1992;149:1028–1032.
17. Ancoli-Israel S, Martin J, Gehrman P, et al. Effect of light on agitation in institutionalized patients with severe Alzheimer disease. *Am J Geriatr Psychiatry.* 2003;11:194–203.
18. Singer C, Hughes R. Clinical use of bright light in geriatric neuropsychiatry. *Lighting for Aging Vision and Health.* LRI-1995. 1995: 143–146.
19. Cooper B, Ward M, Gowland C, McIntosh J. The use of the Lanthony New Color Test in determining the effects of aging on color vision. *J Gerontol.* 1991;46:320–324.
20. Nguyen-Tri D, Overbury O, Faubert J. The role of lenticular senescence in age-related color vision changes. *Invest Ophthalmol Vis Sci.* 2003;44:3698–3704.
21. Cooper B. Long-term care design: current research on the use of color. *J Healthcare Des.* 1993;6:61–67.
22. Adams PF, Marano MA. *Vital Health Statistics: Current Estimates from the National Health Interview Survey, 1994.* Hyattsville, MD: National Center for Health Statistics; 1995;193(Series 10):83–84.
23. Jerger J, Chmiel R, Wilson N, Luchi R. Hearing impairment in older adults: new concepts. *J Am Geriatr Soc.* 1995;43:928–935.
24. Ries, P. W. *Prevalence and Characteristics of Persons With Hearing Trouble: United States, 1990–1991.* Hyattsville, MD: National Center for Health Statistics; 1994;188(Series 10):1–75.
25. National Health Interview Survey—Adults 2008. Retrieved April 2010 from http://www.cdc.gov/nchs/nhis.htm.
26. Cruickshanks KJ, Wiley T L, Tweed TS, et al. Prevalence of hearing loss in older adults in Beaver Dam, Wisconsin. *Am J Epidemiol.* 1998;148:879–886.
27. Hull RH. *Hearing in Aging.* San Diego, CA: Singular; 1995.
28. Cruickshanks KJ, Tweed TS, Wiley TL, et al. The 5-year incidence and progression of hearing loss: the epidemiology of hearing loss study. *Arch Otolaryngol Head Neck Surg.* 2003;129:1041–1046.

29. Hodkinson H. Mental impairment in the elderly. *J Roy Coll Physicians London*. 1973;7:305.
30. Herbst KG, Humphrey C. Hearing impairment and mental state in the elderly living at home. *Br Med J*. 1980;281:903–905.
31. Uhlmann RF, Larson EB, Rees TS, Koepsell TD, Duckert LG. Relationship of hearing impairment to dementia and cognitive dysfunction in older adults. *JAMA*. 1989;261:1916–1919.
32. Schow R, Nerbonne M. Hearing levels among elderly nursing home residents. *J Speech Hear Disord*. 1980;45:124–132.
33. Voeks S, Gallagher C, Langer E, Drinka P. Hearing loss in the nursing home: an institutional issue. *J Am Geriatr Soc*. 1990;38: 141–145.
34. Weinstein BE, Amsel L. Hearing loss and senile dementia in the institutionalized elderly. *Clin Gerontol*. 1986;4:3–15.
35. Gold M, Lightfoot LA, Hnath-Chisolm T. Hearing loss in a memory disorders clinic: an especially vulnerable population. *Arch Neurol*. 1996;53:922–928.
36. Gates GA, Cobb JL, Linn RT, Rees T, Wolf PA, D'Agostino RB. Central auditory dysfunction, cognitive dysfunction, and dementia in older people. *Arch Otolaryngol Head Neck Surg*. 1996; 122:161–167.
37. Ohta RJ, Carlin MR, Harmon BM. Auditory acuity and performance on the mental status questionnaire in the elderly. *J Am Geriatr Soc*. 1981;27:476–478.
38. Uhlmann RF, Larson EB, Koepsell TD. Hearing impairment and cognitive decline in senile dementia of the Alzheimer's type. *J Am Geriatr Soc*. 1986;34:207–210.
39. Allen NH, Burns A, Newton V, et al. The effects of improving hearing in dementia. *Age Aging*. 2003;32:189–193.
40. Kreeger JL, Raulin ML, Grace J, Priest BL. Effect of hearing enhancement on mental status ratings in geriatric psychiatric patients. *Am J Psychiatry*. 1995;152:629–631.
41. Palmer CV, Adams SW, Bourgeois M, Durrant J, Rossi M. Reduction in caregiver-identified problem behaviors in patients with Alzheimer disease post-hearing-aid fitting. *J Speech Lang Hear Res*. 1999;42:312–328.
42. Palmer CV, Adams SW, Durrant JD, Bourgeois M, Rossi M. Managing hearing loss in a patient with Alzheimer's disease. *J Am Acad Audiol*. 1998;9:275–284.
43. Mahendra N, Bayles KA, Harris FP. Effect of presentation modality on immediate and delayed recall in individuals with Alzheimer's disease. *Am J Speech-Lang Pathol*. 2005;14:144–155.

44. Ventry IM, Weinstein BE. Identification of elderly people with hearing problems. *ASHA*. 1983;25:37–42.
45. Belleville S, Peretz I, Malenfant D. Examination of the working memory components in normal aging and in dementia of the Alzheimer type. *Neuropsychologia*. 1996;34:195–207.
46. Cherry BJ, Buckwalter JG, Henderson VW. Memory span procedures in Alzheimer's disease. *Neuropsychology*. 1996;10:286–293.
47. Daneman M, Carpenter PA. Individual differences in working memory and reading. *J Verb Learn Verb Behav*. 1980;19:450–466.
48. Wechsler D. *Wechsler Memory Scale–Third Edition*. San Antonio, TX: Harcourt Assessment; 1997.
49. Anderson JR, Bower GH. *Human Associative Memory*. Washington, DC: Winston; 1972.
50. Hasher L, Zacks RT. Automatic and effortful processes in memory. *J Exp Psych Gen*. 1979;108:356–388.
51. Kintsch W. Models for free recall and recognition. In: Norman DA, ed., *Models of Human Memory*. New York, NY: Academic Press; 1970:333–374.
52. Bayles KA, Tomoeda CK, Kaszniak AW, Trosset MW. Alzheimer's disease effects on semantic memory: loss of structure or function. *J Cogn Neurosci*. 1991;3:166–182.
53. Baddeley AD, Wilson BA. When implicit learning fails: amnesia and the problem of error elimination. *Neuropsychologia*. 1994;32:53–68.
54. Ehlhardt LA, Sohlberg MM, Kennedy M, et al. Evidence-based practice guidelines for instructing individuals with acquired memory impairments: what have we learned in the past 20 years? *Neuropsych Rehab*. 2008;18:300–342.
55. Clare L, Jones RSP. Errorless learning in the rehabilitation of memory impairment: a critical review. *Neuropscyh Rev*. 2008;18: 1–23.
56. Clare L, Wilson BA, Carter G, Breen K, Gosses A, Hodges JR. Intervening with everyday memory problems in dementia of Alzheimer type: an errorless learning approach. *J Clin Exp Neuropsych*. 2000;22:132–146.
57. Wilson BA, Baddeley A, Evans J, Shiel A. Errorless learning in the rehabilitation of memory-impaired people. *Neuropsych Rehab*. 1994;4:307–326.
58. Winter J, Hunkin NM. Re-learning in Alzheimer's disease. *Int J Geriatr Psychiatry*. 1999;14:988–990.
59. Fontaine F. *Apprentissage de nouvelles connaissances chez les patients Alzheimer* [Acquisition of new knowledge in Alzheimer

patients]. Unpublished doctoral dissertation, Université de Montreal; 1995.

60. Wilson BA, Moffat N. The development of group memory therapy. In: Wilson BA, Moffat N, eds, *Clinical Management of Memory Problems.* London, UK: Chapman & Hall; 1992:243–273.
61. Glisky EL, Schacter DL, Tulving E. Learning and retention of computer-related vocabulary in memory-impaired patients: method of vanishing cues. *J Clin Exp Neuropsych.* 1986;8:292–312.
62. Leng NRC, Copello AG, Sayegh A. Learning after brain injury by the method of vanishing cues: a case study. *Behav Psychother.* 1991;19:173–181.
63. Van der Linden M, Coyette F. Acquisition of word processing knowledge in an amnesic patient: implications for theory and rehabilitation. In: Campbell R, Conway M, eds, *Broken Memories: Neuropsychological Case Studies.* Oxford, UK: Blackwell; 1995: 54–80.
64. Bayles KA, Tomoeda CK. *Functional Linguistic Communication Inventory.* Austin, TX: Pro-Ed; 1994.
65. Tulving E, Thomson DM. Encoding specificity and retrieval processes in episodic memory. *Psychological Review.* 1973;80:352–373.
66. Diesfeldt HFA. The importance of encoding instructions and retrieval cues in the assessment of memory in senile dementia. *Arch Gerontol Geriatr.* 1984;3:51–57.
67. Herlitz A, Viitanen M. Semantic organization and verbal episodic memory in patients with mild and moderate Alzheimer's disease. *J Clin Exp Neuropsych.* 1991;13:559–574.
68. Karlsson T, Bäckman L, Herlitz A, Nilsson LG, Winblad B, Österlind PO. Memory improvement at different stages of Alzheimer's disease. *Neuropsychologia.* 1989;27:737–742.
69. Birren JE, Woods A, Williams MV. Behavioral slowing with age: causes, organization, and consequences. In: Poon L, ed, *Aging in the 1980s.* Washington, DC: American Psychological Association; 1980:293–308.
70. Duchek JM, Hunt L, Ball K, Buckles V, Morris JC. The role of selective attention in driving and dementia of the Alzheimer type. *Alzh Dis Assoc Disord.* 1997;11(suppl 1):48–56.
71. Perry RJ, Watson P, Hodges JR. The nature and staging of attention dysfunction in early (minimal and mild) Alzheimer's disease: relationship to episodic and semantic memory impairment. *Neuropsychologia.* 2000;38:252–271.
72. Just MA, Carpenter PA, Keller TA, Emery L, Zajac H, Thulborn

KR. Interdependence of nonoverlapping cortical systems in dual cognitive tasks. *NeuroImage*. 2001;14:417–426.

73. Rees G, Frith CD, Lavie N. Modulating irrelevant motion perception by varying attentional load in an unrelated task. *Science*. 1997;278:1616–1619.

74. Vandenberghe R, Duncan J, Dupont P, et al. Attention to one or two features in left or right visual field: a positron emission tomography study. *J Cogn Neurosci*. 1997;9:419–432.

75. Filoteo JV, Delis DC, Massman PJ, Demadura T, Butters N, Salmon DP. Directed and divided attention in Alzheimer's disease: impairment in shifting attention to global and local stimuli. *J Clin Exp Neuropsych*. 1992;14:871–883.

76. Camicioli R, Howieson D, Lehman S, Kaye J. Talking while walking: the effect of a dual task in aging and Alzheimer's disease. *Neurology*. 1997;48:955–958.

77. Newman SD, Keller TA, Just MA. Volitional control of attention and brain activation in dual task performance. *Human Brain Map*. 2007;28:109–117.

78. Ophir E, Nass C, Wagner AD. Cognitive control in media multitaskers. *Proc Nat Acad Sci U S A*. 2009;106:15583–15587.

79. Perlmuter LC, Monty RA. Motivation and aging. In: Poon L, Rubin DC, Wilson BA, eds, *Everyday Cognition in Adulthood and Late Life*. Cambridge, UK: Cambridge University Press; 1989: 373–393.

80. Pessoa L. How do emotion and motivation direct executive function? *Trends Cogn Sci*. 2009;13:160–166.

81. Vuilleumier P. How brains beware: neural mechanisms of emotional attention. *Trends Cogn Sci*. 2005;9:585–594.

82. Darwin C. *The Expression of the Emotions in Man and Animals*. London, UK: Murray; 1872.

83. Damasio AR. *The Feeling of What Happens: Body and Emotion in the Making of Consciousness*. New York, NY: Harcourt, Brace; 1999.

84. Emery VOB. Retrophylogenesis. In: Emery VOB, Oxman TE, eds, *Dementia*. Baltimore, MD: Johns Hopkins University Press; 2003:177–236.

85. Comblain C, D'Argembeau A, Van der Linden M. Phenomenal characteristics of autobiographical memories for emotional and neutral events in older and younger adults. *Exp Aging Res*. 2005;31:173–189.

86. Haj ME, Postal V, Allain P. Music enhances autobiographical memory in mild Alzheimer's disease. *Ed Gerontol*. 2012;38:30–41.

87. Schaefer A, Philippot P. Selective effects of emotion on the phe-

nomenal characteristics of autobiographical memories. *Memory*. 2005;13:148–160.

88. Talarico JM, LaBar KS, Rubin DC. Emotional intensity predicts autobiographical memory experience. *Mem Cogn*. 2004;32:1118–1132.

89. LaBar KS, Mesulam MM, Gitelman DR, Weintraub S. Emotional curiosity: modulation of visuospatial attention by arousal is preserved in aging and early-stage Alzheimer's disease. *Neuropsychologia*. 2000;38:1734–1740.

90. Moayeri SE, Cahill L, Jin Y, Potkin SG. Relative sparing of emotionally influenced memory in Alzheimer's disease. *NeuroReport*. 2000;11:643–645.

91. Cuddy LL, Duffin J. Music, memory, and Alzheimer's disease: is music recognition spared in dementia, and how can it be assessed? *Med Hypoth*. 2005;645:229–235.

92. Foster NA, Valentine ER. The effect of auditory stimulation on autobiographical recall in dementia. *Exp Aging Res*. 2001; 27:215–228.

93. Irish M, Cunningham CJ, Walsh JB, et al. Investigating the enhancing effect of music on autobiographical memory in mild Alzheimer's disease. *Dement Geriatr Cogn Disord*. 2006;22:108–120.

94. Ochsner KN, Chiu C-YP, Schacter DL. Varieties of priming. *Curr Biol*. 1994;4:189–194.

95. Tulving E, Schacter DL. Priming and human memory systems. *Science*. 1990;247:301–306.

96. Storms LH. Apparent backward association: a situational effect. *J Exp Psych*. 1958;55:390–395.

97. Cofer CN. Experimental studies of the role of verbal processes in concept formation and problem solving. *Ann N Y Acad Sci*. 1960;91:94–107.

98. Halle JW, Spradlin JE. Identifying stimulus control of challenging behavior. In: Reichle J, Wacker DW, eds, *Communicative Alternatives to Challenging Behavior: Integrating Functional Assessment and Intervention Strategies*. Baltimore, MD: Paul H. Brookes; 1993:83–109.

99. Ylvisaker M, Feeney T. Executive functions, self-regulation, and learned optimism in pediatric rehabilitation: a review and implications for intervention. *Pediatr Rehab*. 2002;5:51–70.

100. Bourgeois MS. Enhancing conversation skills in patients with Alzheimer's disease using a prosthetic memory aid. *J Appl Behav Anal*. 1990;23:29–42.

101. Bourgeois MS. Communication treatment for adults with dementia. *J Speech Hear Res*. 1991;34:831–844.
102. Bourgeois MS. Evaluating memory wallets in conversations with persons with dementia. *J Speech Hear Res*. 1992;35:1344–1357.
103. Cuddy LL, Duffin JM, Gill SS, Brown CL, Sikka R, Vanstone AD. Memory for melodies and lyrics in Alzheimer's disease. *Mus Percept*. 2012;29:479–491.
104. Vanstone AD, Cuddy LL, Duffin JM, Alexander E. Exceptional preservation for memory for tunes and lyrics: case studies of amusia, profound deafness and Alzheimer's disease. *Ann N Y Acad Sci*. 2009;1169:291–294.
105. Omar R, Hailstone JC, Warren JD. Semantic memory for music in dementia. *Mus Percept*. 2012;29:467–477.
106. Mahendra N. Manipulation of working memory through sensory stimulation. In: Bayles KA, Hopper T, Mahendra N, Cleary S, Tomoeda CK, eds, *What Works With Dementia Patients and Why*. Short course presented at the American Speech-Language-Hearing Association Convention, San Francisco, CA, November 1999.
107. Mahendra N. Direct interventions for improving the performance of individuals with Alzheimer's disease. *Semin Speech Lang*. 2001;22:291–304.
108. Martin G, Pear J. *Behavior Modification. What It Is and How to Do It*. Upper Saddle River, NJ: Prentice-Hall; 1996.
109. Engelkamp J, Zimmer HD. Memory for action events: a new field of research. *Psych Res*. 1989;51:153–157.
110. Deweer B, Pillon B, Michon A, Dubois F. Mirror reading in Alzheimer's disease: normal skill learning and acquisition of item-specific information. *J Clin Exp Neuropsych*. 1993;15:789–804.
111. Dick MB. Motor and procedural memory in Alzheimer's disease. In: Bäckman L, ed, *Memory Functioning in Dementia*. Amsterdam: North-Holland; 1992:135–150.
112. Zanetti O, Binetti G, Magni E, Rozzini L, Bianchetti A, Trabucchi M. Procedural memory stimulation in Alzheimer's disease: impact of a training program. *Acta Neurol Scand*. 1997;95:152–157.
113. Zanetti O, Zanieri G, Di Giovanni G, et al. Effectiveness of procedural memory stimulation in mild Alzheimer's disease patients. A controlled study. *Neuropsych Rehab*. 2001;11:263–272.
114. Slamecka NJ, Graf P. The generation effect: delineation of a phenomenon. *Human Learn Mem*. 1978;4:592–604.

115. Mitchell DB, Hunt RR, Schmitt FA. The generation effect and reality monitoring: evidence from dementia and normal aging. *J Gerontol.* 1986;41:79–84.

116. Lipinska B, Bäckman L, Mäntylä T, Viitanen M. Effectiveness of self-generated cues in early Alzheimer's disease. *J Clin Exp Neuropsych.* 1994;16:809–816.

117. Millet X, Le Goff M, Bouisson J, Dartigues J-F, Amieva H. Encoding processes influence word-stem completion priming in Alzheimer's disease: a meta-analysis. *J Clin Exp Neuropsych.* 2010;32:494–504.

118. Thornton S, Brotchie J. Reminiscence: a critical review of the empirical literature. *Brit J Clin Psych.* 1987;26:93–111.

119. Hellen CR. *Alzheimer's Disease: Activity-focused Care.* Newton, MA: Butterworth-Heinemann; 1992.

120. Sheridan C. Reminiscence. In: Alzheimer's Association, ed, *Activity Programming for Persons With Dementia: A Sourcebook.* Chicago, IL: The Alzheimer's Association; 1995.

121. Gillies C, James A. *Reminiscence Work With Old People.* London, UK: Chapman & Hall; 1994.

122. Boczko F. The Breakfast Club: a multi-modal language stimulation program for nursing home residents with Alzheimer's disease. *Am J Alzh Care Rel Disord Res.* 1994;9:35–38.

123. Kliegl R, Smith J, Baltes PB. Testing-the-limits of the study of adult age differences in cognitive plasticity of a mnemonic skill. *Dev Psych.* 1989;25:247–256.

124. Verhaeghen P, Marcoen A, Goossens L. Improving memory performance in the aged through mnemonic training: a meta-analytic study. *Psych Aging.* 1992;7:242–251.

125. Yesavage JA, Rose TL, Bower GH. Interactive imagery and affective judgments improve face-name learning in the elderly. *J Gerontol.* 1983;38:197–203.

126. Bäckman L, Small B. Influences of cognitive support on episodic remembering: tracing the process of loss from normal aging to Alzheimer's disease. *Psych Aging.* 1998;13:267–276.

127. Bird M, Luszcz M. Encoding specificity, depth of processing, and cued recall in Alzheimer's disease. *J Clin Exp Neuropsych.* 1991;13:508–520.

128. Arkin SM, Rose C, Hopper T. Implicit and explicit learning gains in Alzheimer's patients: effects of naming and information retrieval training. *Aphasiology.* 2000;14:723–742.

129. Glasgow RE, Zeiss RA, Barrera M, Lewinshon PM. Case studies on remediating memory deficits in brain-injured patients. *J Clin Psych.* 1977;33:1049–1054.

130. Van der Linden M, Van der Kaa MM. Reorganization therapy for memory impairments. In: Seron X, Deloche G, eds, *Cognitive Approaches in Neuropsychological Rehabilitation*. Hillsdale, NJ: Lawrence Erlbaum Associates; 1989:105–158.
131. Stevens A, King CA, Camp CJ. Improving prose memory and social interaction using question asking reading with adult day care clients. *Ed Gerontol*. 1993;19:651–662.
132. McCarthy DL. Investigation of a visual imagery mnemonic device for acquiring name-face associations. *J Exp Psych Human Learn Mem*. 1980;6:145–155.
133. Green RL. *Human Memory: Paradigms and Paradoxes*. Hillsdale, NJ: Lawrence Erlbaum Associates; 1992.
134. Glisky EL. Rehabilitation and memory disorders: tapping into preserved mechanisms. *Brain Cogn*. 1997;35:291–292.
135. Heun R, Burkart M, Benkert O. Improvement of picture recall by repetition in patients with dementia of the Alzheimer type. *Int J Geriatr Psychiatry*. 1997;12:85–92.
136. Little AG, Volans PJ, Hemsley DR, Levy R. The retention of new information in senile dementia. *Brit J Clin Psych*. 1986;25:71–72.
137. Small JA, Kemper S, Lyons K. Sentence comprehension in Alzheimer's disease: effects of grammatical complexity, speech rate, and repetition. *Psych Aging*. 1997;12:3–11.
138. Brush JA, Camp CJ. *A Therapy Technique for Improving Memory: Spaced Retrieval*. Beachwood, OH: Authors; 1998.
139. Schacter DL, Rich SA, Stampp M. S. Remediation of memory disorders: An experimental evaluation of the spaced retrieval technique. *J Clin Exp Neuropsych*. 1985;7:79–96.
140. Landauer TK, Bjork RA. Optimum rehearsal patterns and name learning. In Gruneberg MM, Morriss PE, Sykes RN, eds, *Practical Aspects of Memory*. New York, NY: Academic Press; 1978:625–632.
141. Abrahams JP, Camp CJ. Maintenance and generalization of object naming training in anomia associated with degenerative dementia. *Clin Gerontol*. 1993;12:57–72.
142. Camp CJ. Facilitation of new learning in Alzheimer's disease. In Gilmore GC, Whitehouse PJ, Wykle ML, eds, *Memory, Aging and Dementia*. New York, NY: Springer; 1989:212–225.
143. Camp CJ, & Schaller J. Epilogue: Spaced-retrieval memory training in an adult day-care center. *Educational Gerontology*, 1989; 15: 641–648.
144. Moffat, NJ. Home-based cognitive rehabilitation with the elderly. In: Poon L, Rubin DC, Wilson BA, eds, *Everyday Cognition*

in Adulthood and Late Life. Cambridge, UK: Cambridge University Press; 1989:659–690.

145. Vanhalle C, Van der Linden M, Belleville S, Gilbert B. Putting names on faces: use of spaced retrieval strategy in a patient with dementia of Alzheimer type. American Speech Language & Hearing Association, Special Interest Division 2 Newsletter. *Neurophysiol Neurogenic Speech Lang Disord.* 1998;8:17–21.

146. Jacquemin A, Van der Linden M, Feyereisen P. Thérapie du manque du mot chez un patient bilingue présentant une maladie d'Alzheimer probable. *Questions de Logopédie.* 1993;27:91–96.

147. McKitrick LA, Camp CJ. Relearning the names of things: the spaced retrieval intervention implemented by caregivers. *Clin Gerontol.* 1993;14:60–62.

148. Moffat, N. Strategies of memory therapy. In: Wilson BA, Moffat N, eds, *Clinical Management of Memory Problems.* 2nd ed. London, UK: Chapman & Hall; 1992:86–119.

149. Bird MJ. Psychosocial rehabilitation for problems arising from cognitive deficits in dementia. In: Hill RD, Bäckman L, Stigsdotter-Neely A, eds, *Cognitive Rehabilitation in Old Age.* New York, NY: Oxford University Press; 2000:249–267.

150. Camp CJ, Bird MJ, Cherry KE. Retrieval strategies as a rehabilitation aid for cognitive loss in pathological aging. In: Hill RD, Bäckman L, Stigsdotter-Neely A, eds, *Cognitive Rehabilitation in Old Age.* New York, NY: Oxford University Press; 2000:224–248.

151. Brush JA, Camp CJ. Using spaced-retrieval as an intervention during speech-language therapy. *Clin Gerontol.* 1998;19:51–64.

152. Davis RN, Massman PJ, Doody RS. Cognitive intervention in Alzheimer's disease: a randomized placebo-controlled study. *Alzh Dis Assoc Disord.* 2001;15:1–9.

153. Erkes J, Raffard S, Meulemans T. Spaced-retrieval in patients with Alzheimer's disease: critical review and clinical applications. *Psychologie Neuropsychiatrie du Vieillissement.* 2009;7: 275–286.

Unit 8

Treatment: Indirect Interventions

Indirect interventions, the focus of this unit, include linguistic modifications that facilitate communication with individuals with dementia, computer supports, memory aids that improve quality of life, and environmental manipulations. Speech-language pathologists do not carry out indirect interventions but recommend them in care plans, teach them to caregivers, and oversee their implementation. Medicare will pay for the development of functional maintenance care plans and caregiver training.

Linguistic Modifications

Numerous linguistic modifications help dementia patients communicate by facilitating cognitive processing. They can be classified according to their impact on language comprehension and production.

Improving Language Comprehension

Language comprehension is a complex, multistage process.[1] Listeners must analyze the form, content, and context in which an utterance is spoken to derive the proposition(s) being expressed. Thus, techniques for facilitating comprehension can be subcategorized according to whether they primarily involve the form, content, or use of language.

Form

Use a Slower Than Normal Rate of Speech. As previously mentioned, the brain damage associated with dementing diseases results in slower information processing, as does normal aging. By slowing speech rate, the load on memory is reduced because the greater the number of words spoken per minute, the more concepts the individual must process. The average rate of speech is 160 to 170 words per minute, but fast speakers produce 200 or more words per minute. Calculate your normal rate of speech, and if you are a fast speaker, slow your rate to slightly less than average.

Provide Multimodal Input. Learning and comprehension are better when information is experienced in more than one modality. Hearing information and being able to review it in written form is better than simply hearing it because of the rapid forgetting that characterizes many types of dementia. Providing information in one sensory modality and then another also capitalizes on the value of repetition for strengthening encoding. For example, to teach a name, it is better to explain the name, show the patient its written form, then have the patient read the name, write the name, and associate it with a face or picture that can be described.

Because Alzheimer's dementia (AD) patients retain the ability to read words far into the course of the disease, it is generally helpful to use the visual modality in addition to the auditory modality for providing information. Similarly, because they have difficulty holding information in mind, it is better to provide the object being discussed.[2]

Limit the Number of Conversational Partners. Keeping track of the topic, and who said what to whom, when several people are conversing can overwhelm dementia patients because of deficits in attention and memory.[3,4] Many caregivers fail to appreciate this fact and are surprised when the dementia patient becomes agitated at large family gatherings. Dementia patients do best communicating one on one.

Use a Pleasant, Accepting Vocal Tone. Everyone becomes uncomfortable when someone speaks in an unfriendly tone. Even dementia patients, who no longer have the capacity to process word meaning, respond to the prosodic and emotional characteristics of speech. Clinicians and caregivers who use an accepting vocal tone evoke a positive reaction from the patient. People who use a condescending or threatening tone create emotional distress that interferes with comprehension.

Content

Reduce the Number of Propositions in Sentences. The greater the number of propositions, the more cognitive resources listeners must garner to interpret and act on the message. Rochon et al[1] administered a battery of working memory and sentence comprehension tests to AD patients and age- and education-matched elders. Individuals with AD were found to have reduced spans and impaired central executive processes. Rochon and colleagues observed that the number of propositions in stimulus sentences affected the performance of AD patients. When sentences contained a single proposition, AD patients performed like normal elders; when they contained 2 propositions, AD patients' performance was significantly inferior to that of normal elders. By simplifying syntax, the number of propositions can be reduced. Consider the differences in cognitive demand of the following sentences.

1. One proposition: The man arrived late.
2. Two propositions: The man, who was coming from Memphis to Little Rock, arrived late. (*proposition 1: man was late; proposition 2: the man was coming from Memphis to Little Rock*)
3. Three propositions: He was traveling from Memphis to Little Rock on a recently refurbished airplane that took off late. (*proposition 1: he was traveling from Memphis to Little Rock; proposition 2: the airplane was recently refurbished; proposition 3: the airplane took off late*)
4. Four propositions: The airplane that was coming from Memphis was late, but the airplane that was coming from Phoenix was early. (*proposition 1: the airplane was late; proposition 2: the airplane was coming from Memphis; proposition 3: the airplane was early; proposition 4: the airplane was coming from Phoenix*)

Simple subject-verb-object sentences, like sentence 1, require the fewest cognitive resources because they are the least demanding on memory. When embedded clauses are added, as in sentence 2, memory load is increased. Embedded clauses interrupt the main clause (who was coming from Memphis to Little Rock) and the listener must hold part of the main clause (man) in memory while processing the embedded clause (who was coming from Memphis to Little Rock). Sentence 3 contains multiple propositions and embedding. In sentence 4, two main clauses are joined by a conjunction and both contain an embedded relative clause. Four propositions are expressed. Conjoining propositions increases memory load, as does embedding.

Left-branching sentences with an initial dependent clause, such as "When he was traveling from Memphis to Little Rock, he developed air sickness," are harder to process than right-branching sentences, such as "He developed air sickness when he was traveling from Memphis to Little Rock." Dependent clauses occurring before the main clause must be held in mind until the listener/reader comes to the main clause.

Talk About the Here and Now. Because dementia patients have difficulty recalling episodic information, they do best when the conversation concerns something they can see and feel—in other words, something to which they can refer. Doing an activity with the patient provides something to talk about. Many clinicians have observed that patients talk more when doing an activity. Myriad activities like arranging flowers, building an object, sewing, and painting provide a topic for conversation about the here and now.

Simplify Vocabulary. All of us have stronger engrams for simple, high-frequency words than infrequently used words. The same is true for individuals with dementia. Thus, it is important to share information using common, high-frequency words. Although the following sentences A and B express the same meaning, sentence B is easier to comprehend.

A. The philatelist was a centenarian.
B. The stamp collector was a hundred years old.

Replace Pronouns With Proper Nouns. All pronouns have antecedents that must be remembered for pronoun and sentence comprehension. Dementia patients with episodic memory deficits have difficulty remembering antecedents. By repeating the proper noun, rather than using a pronoun, as in the following sentence 2, memory load is reduced and comprehension facilitated.[5]

1. John and Mary went to see Bill before he left for college. They wanted to wish him well.
2. John and Mary went to see Bill before *Bill* left for college. *John and Mary* wanted to wish *Bill* well.

Revise and Restate That Which Was Not Understood. Occasionally, more than one explanation of a phenomenon or event is needed for us to comprehend. All of us know that some explanations are more comprehensible than others. When a dementia patient fails to comprehend, revising and restating the information may improve comprehension, especially if done in a noncondescending way.

Use

Ask Multiple-Choice or Yes/No Questions. Some question forms are less cognitively demanding than others. Open-ended questions like "What did you do last night?" place your conversational partner in a free-recall situation. With a moment's reflection, healthy adults can mentally reconstruct the events of the previous night; however, individuals with AD and other dementias associated with episodic memory impairment cannot. Although questions like "What do you want for dinner?" do not place individuals in a free-recall situation, they nonetheless pose difficulty because they require the generation of possibilities. Generating ideas is another cognitive ability impaired early in dementia. Choice questions like "Would you like chicken or pasta for dinner?" do not place patients in a free-recall situation or require them to generate possibilities; they must simply make a choice. Table 8–1 gives examples of difficult and easier types of questions.

Use Direct Rather Than Indirect Speech Acts. Indirect speech acts are best explained by example. Frequently used ones are where person A says to person B, "Can you pass the sugar?" or "Why can't I ever find the remote control?" In both of these examples, person A *is* making a request of the listener *indirectly* by asking a question. Being indirect is a way of being polite. When people are direct and say, "Pass the sugar" or "Find the remote control," they can be perceived as demanding and rude. Nonetheless, direct statements, politely worded, are often easier for dementia patients to understand, for example, "Please pass the sugar" or "Please help me find the remote control."

Table 8–1. Difficult and Easy Types of Questions

Difficult Types of Questions	Open-Ended Free Recall:	Open-Ended Generative:
	Of the movies you have seen, what is your favorite?	What should we buy Lesley for her birthday?
Easier Types of Questions	**Two-Choices:**	**Yes-No:**
	Would you like Mexican or Chinese food for dinner?	Do you like to travel?
	Do you want to buy Lesley a watch or necklace for her birthday?	Do you want to buy Lesley a watch for her birthday?

Avoid Teasing and Sarcasm. Many forms of teasing and sarcasm involve exaggeration or being nonliteral. For example, the nurse who said, "You look so good today that I'll bet all the girls will be asking you for a date" to a confused nursing home patient was exaggerating. The interpretation of exaggeration, teasing, and sarcasm require sensitivity to context, an activity that is beyond the capacity of many demented individuals.

Avoid Talking to the Patient Like a Child. Talking to the patient like a child is demeaning and provides a poor model for other caregivers. Many patients will be offended even if they are unable to articulate their perceptions.

Try Amplifying the Voice of the Speaker. Many caregivers report the effectiveness of assistive listening devices (Figure 8–1) in communicating with AD patients. Assistive listening devices look similar to a conventional body-worn hearing aid and serve to provide general sound level gain. They improve speech-to-noise ratio and help patients focus their attention.[6] This is especially true if the caregiver has a soft voice.

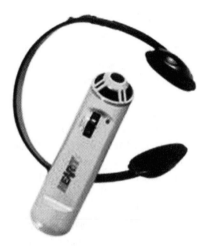

Figure 8–1. Example of an assistive listening device. Photo provided courtesy of Hearit LLC, a division of Speech Banana Therapies, http://www.hearitllc.com.

Improving Production of Language

Provide Something Tangible and/or Visible to Stimulate Conversation

This strategy is similar to talking about the here and now and helps both production and comprehension because it gives the patient and caregiver a point of reference. Furthermore, the apprehension by the patient of the tangible/visible object causes concepts related to the object to be activated through the process of spreading activation. This often results in the patient being able to call to mind other information that can be shared in the conversation. Memory wallets and books containing information about the patient stimulate language production and are an excellent example of this technique. Bourgeois[7] wrote a book about conversing with dementia patients through these memory assistive devices.

Bourgeois[7] has shown that some dementia patients are more likely to make meaningful utterances when a memory wallet or book is the stimulus to conversation. The memory wallet is a compilation of pictures and sentences about the patient's life. The patient does not have to actively recall the pictured events, merely recognize them. Bourgeois observed that pictures and sentences enabled subjects in her studies to recall related information. The memory book is a larger version of the memory wallet. Memory books include biographical information and facts about people important to the patient that have been simply stated and paired with pictures and other memorabilia.

According to Bourgeois, mild dementia patients, those who score 19 to 24 on the Mini-Mental State Examination (MMSE), receive excellent benefit from the wallets and books. Then, too, mild patients are aware that they have the wallets and books and refer to them on their own. Moderately impaired patients, whose MMSE scores range between 12 and 18, typically require caregiver prompting to use the aids. Severely demented individuals, whose MMSE scores are lower than 12, may not benefit from the aids.

Hopper et al[2] used a single-subject experimental design with replications across subjects to investigate the efficacy of using dolls and stuffed animals to stimulate meaningful communication in 4 females with AD who were moderately demented. Study participants produced more relevant information units when the dolls and stuffed animals were used as conversational stimuli than when questions alone were used. Also, the AD patients clearly enjoyed the dolls and stuffed animals, as evident by their increased animation when they were presented and their hugging and talking to them.

Provide Food to Increase Sociability and Talking Among Patients

Refreshments create a social atmosphere and are a cultural trigger for conversation. Many long-term care facilities have programs in which residents gather daily to make breakfast and talk about world events (Figure 8–2). One program called The Breakfast Club has been described by Boczko[8] and Santo Pietro and Boczko.[9] Others have afternoon teatime. Many dementia patients enjoy preparing food and if done with supervision, food preparation can be a useful and pleasurable stimulus for socialization and conversation.

Avoid Placing Patients in a Free-Recall Situation

Recently we visited a patient and caregiver at home. Both greeted us at the door and the caregiver said, "You remember Cheryl and Kathryn, dear, they are here to test your memory." The patient

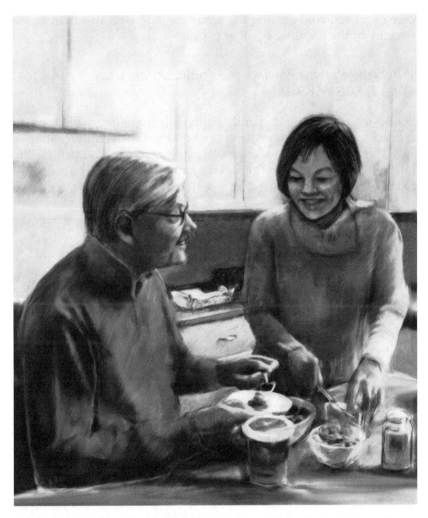

Figure 8–2. Providing refreshments or serving a meal creates a social context for communication. Photo courtesy of the National Institute of Diabetes and Digestive and Kidney Disease, National Institutes of Health, Image N01164.

responded, "Oh, yes, nice to see you again." Had the caregiver not provided our names and explained the purpose of our visit, the patient would have floundered and been embarrassed. The sensitivity of this caregiver to her spouse's inability to freely recall our names and appointment preserved his dignity. Clinicians should counsel caregivers to avoid placing the patient in a free-recall situation, especially in the presence of other people.

When the Patient Forgets the Topic, Summarize What Has Been Said

A classic problem for dementia patients is forgetting what they intended to say, thereby causing the communicative interchange to fail. The thoughtful listener can summarize what has been said to enable the patient to continue. This strategy helps the patient save face. The following is an example of the benefit of this strategy.

> *Context*: An individual with dementia and her friend were talking during lunch that consisted of salad.
> *Patient*: I used to have a garden and raise tomatoes. We would go out to the garden with a salt shaker you know and . . . [here the patient forgot what she was going to say] let me see, oh my, uh . . .
> *Caregiver*: Going to the tomato garden with a salt shaker was a good way to get a snack.
> *Patient*: Yes, we picked tomatoes and ate them right in the garden.

If the Patient Wishes to Write a Letter, Supply the Materials, a List of News Items, and a Picture of the Letter's Intended Recipient

This type of support makes it easier for the patient to be successful in producing a letter. Even healthy adults have trouble thinking of things to write. Having a few news items written down eliminates the need for the patient to remember and may stimulate related memories. Also, being able to see the person for whom the letter is intended sharpens the patient's focus.

Have the Patient Read Aloud

Because the mechanics of reading remain intact for many patients late into the disease course, this is a language production activity they can do. One caregiver friend of ours had her husband read popular novels aloud while she worked in the kitchen preparing food. He felt useful and she enjoyed the stories. We have heard many reports of elders with dementia who read story-books to children in day care centers or their own grandchildren.

Do Not Repeatedly Correct the Patient

Dementia patients often make erroneous statements, and too often, caregivers embarrass them by correcting misinformation, particularly when other people are present. Once a patient has been put on the defensive, agitation and hostility may result, and he or she loses the desire to talk.

A strategy for indirectly correcting a patient with an erroneous idea is to provide the correct information in the patient's memory wallet or scrapbook. Frequent use of the wallet or book may help the patient stay informed. One moderately demented AD patient repeatedly told caregivers that her son was coming home from school, and she needed to make supper. The caregiver put her son's picture in his Navy uniform on her nightstand and every day reviewed the fact of his being at sea. In a few days, the patient's confusion about her son's whereabouts diminished, and she told people that her son was in the Navy.

Computer Supports

Computer-Based Assistive Technology

Advances in computer technology are increasingly being used to support the functioning of cognitively and communicatively impaired individuals. "Cognitive prostheses" or "cognitive orthoses" are collectively known as ATC, or assistive technology for cognition.[10] ATC interventions are extrinsic environmental supports for orientation, prospective memory, communication, executive functioning, and activities of daily living (ADLs). They can provide reminders, cue and monitor performance, alert caregivers to problems, expose patients to virtual environments, stimulate communication, and help people compensate for sensory loss. Although the application of ATCs to the treatment of individuals with progressive dementia is still in its infancy, reports to date are encouraging, especially regarding prospective memory aids (see LoPresti et al[10] for a review).

In several places in Europe, elders with no previous computer experience are using flat, touchscreen computers to obtain reminders about how to do basic tasks, stay oriented, and Skype with family.[11] These systems also have a means of sharing information that enable family members to check on loved ones. Computers are also being used to stimulate cognition and entertain. Individuals with mild AD who received 24 weeks of computer-based cognitive stimulation plus psychostimulation had improved outcome scores on the MMSE and the Alzheimer's Disease Assessment Scale–Cognitive compared with those who had only psychostimulation.[12] Many apps for game playing and stimulation are being used by individuals with mild to moderate dementia; for example, patients are playing a simplified version of scrabble on iPads with friends. The iPad touchscreen and intuitive operations are within the capacity of many dementia patients.

Robots

Robot and computer technology are linked and a variety of robots have been developed to assist elders. They can be programmed with information about the elder's daily activities and have the capacity to provide needed reminders.[13] Also their sensing systems can detect problems and alert caregivers. Sensors make it possible to locate misplaced objects that are radiofrequency identification tagged. They can also be programmed to call 911 if no movement by the patient is observed. A robot named Gerry was developed that is basically Skype on wheels.[14] Its mobility and ease of use enable dementia patients to Skype with loved ones and have been reported to enhance mood and quality of life. Robotic animals are being widely used to provide social stimulation to dementia patients of all levels of severity.[15] Best known is Paro the baby harp seal, which responds to touch and sound and is capable of learning the patterns of response of the individuals who interact with it. Wada[16] reported that 20 minutes with Paro increased cortical neuronal activity significantly. Mordoch and colleagues[15] provide an excellent review of the literature on the use of social commitment robots in the care of elders with dementia. In fact, there are many reports of the positive response of nursing home residents to Paro and other robotic animals who increase social interaction and elevate mood.[17–20]

Prompting System

A multidisciplinary team in Scotland designed a conversation support and prompting system for people with dementia.[21] The system uses touchscreen technology to access a multimedia reminiscence presentation that prompts conversation. The rationale for the system's development is the difficulty that dementia patients have conversing because of deficits in the ability to freely recall information and events. The conversation support system compensates for that difficulty. It provides information that dementia patients have difficulty recalling but retain in long-term memory, thereby stimulating reminiscence. Results of a pilot study show that the reminiscence presentation system maintains the interest of individuals with dementia, is easy to use, and gives the patient control over the communication interaction. Staff and family members also responded positively to the system, and modifications are under way to increase the quantity and quality of systems prompts.

Prospective Memory Aids

Many prospective memory aids are commercially available. Most are pocket-sized devices that can record and play back verbal messages. They contain software that stores a schedule (and in some cases, other information), and sophisticated models can send and receive information. These aids can signal users to do scheduled things through auditory and/or visual cues. Zanetti et al[22] studied the ability of mild and moderate AD patients to use a prospective memory aid, specifically an electronic agenda. Five subjects were given 7 memory tasks to complete at fixed times over the course of a day. Task completion with and without the device was compared. When the electronic agenda was available, task completion significantly improved and 2 of the subjects had perfect scores.

Mihailidis et al[23] used artificial intelligence to develop COACH (Cognitive Orthosis for Assisting Activities in the Home), a device to help individuals with dementia complete ADLs. COACH uses artificial intelligence algorithms and a video camera connected to a computer to monitor behavior. For example, it can monitor hand washing and provide prerecorded verbal prompts. Hand washing behavior was tested for 60 days with 10 individuals with moderate to severe dementia. Results showed that the number of hand washing steps completed without caregiver assistance increased by 25% when group data were analyzed. Systems like COACH can support myriad activities.

SenseCam

The SenseCam[24] is designed to make a digital record of the events experienced by the individual wearing it. A small digital camera with a wide-angle lens is worn around the neck and it can be programmed to automatically take photographs at certain times. Also, sensors are built in and monitored by a microprocessor. Certain changes in sensor readings can trigger the taking of a photograph— for example, detection of the body heat of someone near the camera. It is being tested for a variety of uses.

Life Story Work

The development of the life stories of dementia patients is being widely studied as a tool to benefit patients and caregivers, professional and personal. McKeown and colleagues[25] report that development of life stories enables staff to "see" the personhood of the patient and helps patients maintain memory of life events. Thompson[26] reports that life stories stimulate conversation and provide comfort to agitated patients.

A House as a Cognitive Orthotic

Mynatt et al[27] have described their concept of an "instrumented environment" or house. It will have information about the inhabitants' activities and lifestyle and contain sensors that detect task disruptions. Various auditory and visual cuing systems throughout the house will assist inhabitants in the completion of multistep activities (eg, washing clothes, making breakfast, emptying the trash). Finally, the sensors will be used to detect the need for emergency assistance.

Caregiver Counseling Basics

Creating a Safe Environment

The goal of environmental manipulation is the creation of a safe, peaceful, and organized environment that evokes positive mood and behavior. The following suggestions will help achieve safety:

■ Remove guns or other weapons.
■ Lock up poisons, insecticides, solvents, paints, and medications.
■ Put a nightlight in the patient's bedroom and bathroom.
■ Install a safety gate at stairwells.
■ Fasten edges of rugs.
■ Secure sliding glass doors.
■ Place decals on glass doors.
■ Secure electric cords to prevent tripping.
■ Put on door locks that will prevent the patient from wandering away; however, be sure the patient has an exit in the event of fire.
■ Place a sturdy light by the patient's bed with a remote switch.
■ Put nonslip mats in tub and shower areas.
■ Have an identification bracelet made with the patient's name, address, and note about being memory impaired.
■ Give police a current photo or videotape of the patient.
■ Keep an article of worn clothing wrapped tightly in a plastic bag to be used to help track the lost patient.
■ Deter the patient from driving.

A safety issue for individuals with dementia and others is driving. Gilley and colleagues[28] conducted a large study of driving and AD and discovered that the median duration of driving after disease onset was approximately 2 ½ years. Younger drivers and men were less likely to stop driving despite significant cognitive impairment. Twenty-two percent of the AD patients who were driving had been involved in an accident in the previous 6 months. These investigators indicated that patients with MMSE scores of 18 or lower, who showed evidence of visuospatial impairment, were unlikely to be safe drivers. Patients whose MMSE scores are 18 or higher and who have no visuospatial impairment or minimal impairment should be given an in-car driving evaluation to ensure that they can drive safely on familiar routes.

To create peaceful, organized environments that support basic ADLs, consider the following:

- Keep the environment constant.
- Minimize visual distractions.
- Eliminate extraneous noise.
- Remove clutter.
- Keep needed objects visible (eg, comb and brush).
- Remove mirrors (patients may not recognize themselves and become alarmed at the presence of a "stranger").
- Use orientation signs (eg, bathroom, bedroom).
- Display a calendar orienting the patient to the day's events, for example:
  - 9:00 Get newspaper
  - 10:00 Haircut at Sam's Barber Shop
  - 11:00 Grocery store for milk
  - 12:00 Lunch (egg salad sandwich and tomato soup)
  - 1:00 Rest
  - 3:00 Walk in the neighborhood
  - 4:00 Visit from granddaughter Isabella
  - 6:00 Dinner (chicken and rice)
  - Evening Watch TV at home

The physical characteristics of an environment influence how people feel and respond. Each patient's environment should be analyzed in relation to what it evokes in terms of mood, language, and action. This analysis is particularly important for patients who are exhibiting negative behaviors and/or are highly agitated. The following will help create a happy mood and positive behavior:

- Accessible familiar objects
- Pleasant aromas
- Sufficient lighting
- Culturally appropriate decor
- Choice of well-liked foods
- Pictures of past happy events
- An energy outlet space where the patient can safely walk
- Accessible craft materials and work tables
- Music premorbidly preferred
- Opportunities to do common procedures like folding laundry, raking leaves, setting the table
- Regular touching through manicures, hair styling, massage.

Music

Music is a potent tool for engaging patients and stimulating reminiscence. It has been shown to reduce agitation,[29] loneliness, and depression,[30] and stimulate participation in activities.[31] Helmes and Wiancko[32] reported that playing quiet baroque music significantly reduced noisemaking behavior in some dementia patients. Gerdner and Swanson[33] observed that music preferred by dementia patients premorbidly produced a beneficial effect on behavior. Clinicians should obtain information about the music preferences of the patient and provide a means for turning off unwanted music.

Having Something to Nurture

A highly successful approach to designing nursing homes is to provide dementia patients something to nurture—for example, pets and plants. Thomas[34] revolutionized the long-term care industry with his Eden Alternative™ system of care, which he developed in response to the isolation and inactivity he observed in nursing home residents. Thomas advocated for nursing homes to be "human habitats" where residents live, feel useful and needed, and even thrive, as opposed to a place where they go to wait to die. A fundamental principle of the Eden Alternative model calls for residents to be given the opportunity to give as well as receive care. Using this approach, Thomas[34] reported that residents experienced fewer urinary tract infections, a decrease in upper respiratory infections, a decrease in medication use, and fewer deaths. Additionally, use of the Eden Alternative has resulted in decreased staff turnover. Resnick and Ransom[35] documented fewer behavioral incidents and decreased restraint use in Eden nursing homes compared with traditional nursing homes, and Bergman-Evans[36] reported lower levels of boredom and helplessness over a 1-year period in residents of a certified Eden Alternative facility compared with residents of a non-Eden facility.

Supporting Feeding

Speech-language pathologists are frequently asked for help with the challenges of feeding dementia patients. Moderate and severely demented AD patients often require eating assistance. Environmental manipulations can improve functional feeding in many patients, and the following suggestions are based on the observations of Van Ort and Phillips[37]:

- Have the same individual feed the patient.
- Feed the patient in the same place each time.
- Have assistants feed 1 patient at a time.
- Do not allow interruptions during the feeding.
- Position the food so the patient can see it.
- Use finger foods when possible.
- Place a spoon in the patient's hand.
- Provide a model of scooping food and taking it to the mouth.
- Pace feeding so that the time between bites is about the same.
- Avoid mixing and stirring foods.
- Pair touch with the initiation of feeding and use it consistently as a cue.
- Watch for cues from the patient that s/he wants another bite.
- Offer drinks frequently during feeding.
- Eliminate distractions such as a blaring television.
- Provide social reinforcement for feeding such as hugs, touching, and compliments.

Involve the Verbally Repetitious Patient in a Physical Activity to Reduce Perseveration

Admonishing repetitious patients to quit repeating is ineffective because their episodic memory problems cause them to forget admonitions. However, changing the activity, especially to one that is physical, may eliminate the cues that elicit the ideational repetition.

When moderate or late-stage dementia patients produce disruptive vocalizations, such as screaming and repeatedly calling out, it may be a sign that they are experiencing physical discomfort or emotional distress, are understimulated or overstimulated, or have an unmet need.[38] Caregivers should be trained to consider these possibilities. Smith and Filips[39] have an excellent summary of the causes of disruptive vocalizations and strategies to decrease them (http://www.healthcare.uiowa.edu/igec). The following is a short adaptation of their recommended interventions:

- Understimulation: Involve patient in enjoyable activities.
- Overstimulation: Simplify environment, have quiet periods.
- Pain: Reposition, provide exercise, medication.
- Fatigue: Have rest periods.
- Depression: Reduce sources of stress and fear.
- Immobility: Take on outings.
- Psychosis: Minimize sensory input.

Summary of Important Points

- Indirect interventions involve modifying the linguistic and physical environments of individuals with dementia to improve cognitive-communicative functioning and quality of life.
- To improve *linguistic comprehension*, consider:
  - Using a slower than normal rate of speech
  - Providing multimodal input
  - Limiting the number of conversational partners
  - Using a pleasant, accepting vocal tone
  - Reducing the number of propositions in sentences
  - Talking about the here and now
  - Using direct rather than indirect speech acts
  - Avoiding teasing and sarcasm
  - Avoiding talking to the patient like a child
  - Amplifying the voice of the speaker.
- To improve the *production of language*, consider:
  - Providing something tangible and/or visible to stimulate conversation
  - Avoiding placing patients in a free-recall situation
  - Summarizing what has been said when the patient forgets the topic
  - Supplying materials, a list of news items, and a picture of the letter's intended recipient if the patient wants to write a letter
  - Respectfully supplying the word the patient is struggling to remember
  - Having the patient read aloud to the caregiver or together with the caregiver
  - Not repeatedly correcting the patient
  - Engaging patients in activities

- Involve the verbally repetitious patient in a physical activity to reduce perseveration.
- Provide food to increase sociability and talking among patients.
- The goal of environmental manipulation is to create an environment that is safe, peaceful, and organized and that evokes positive mood and behavior.
- Left unoccupied, dementia patients become confused, agitated, and afraid. Thus, while they are awake, involve them in enjoyable activities and provide something for them to nurture.

References

1. Rochon E, Waters GS, Caplan D. The relationship between measures of working memory and sentence comprehension in patients with Alzheimer's disease. *J Speech Lang Hear Res.* 2000; 43:395–413.
2. Hopper T, Bayles KA, Tomoeda CK. Using toys to stimulate communicative function in individuals with Alzheimer's disease. *J Med Speech Lang Pathol.* 1998;6:73–80.
3. Baddeley AD, Baddeley HA, Bucks RS, Wilcock GK. Attentional control in Alzheimer's disease. *Brain.* 2001;124:1492–1508.
4. Collette F, Van der Linden BM, Salmon E. Phonological loop and central executive functioning in Alzheimer's disease. *Neuropsychologia.* 1999;37:905–918.
5. Almor A, Kempler D, MacDonald MC, Andersen ES, Tyler LK. Why do Alzheimer patients have difficulty with pronouns? Working memory, semantics, and reference in comprehension and production in Alzheimer's disease. *Brain Lang.* 1999; 67:202–227.
6. Doherty KA, Brangman SA. Improving communication for older hospital patients with assistive listening devices. *Update,* SUNY Upstate Medical University; 2011:2,6.
7. Bourgeois MS. *Conversing With Memory Impaired Individuals Using Memory Aids.* Gaylord, MI: Northern Speech Services; 1992.
8. Boczko F. The Breakfast Club: a multi-modal language stimulation program for nursing home residents with Alzheimer's disease. *Am J Alzh Dis Other Dement.* 1994;9:35–38.
9. Santo Pietro MJ, Boczko F. Breakfast Club: results of a study examining the effectiveness of a multi-modality group communication treatment. *Am J Alzh Dis Other Dement.* 1998;13:146–158.

10. LoPresti EF, Mihailidis A, Kirsch N. Assistive technology for cognitive rehabilitation: state of the art. *Neuropsych Rehab.* 2004;14:5–39.
11. Technology for people living with dementia. Euronews, Sci-Tech/Futuris Web site. Retrieved November 2010 from http://www.euronews.com/2010/04/11/technology-for-people-living-with-dementia/.
12. Tárraga L, Boada M, Modinos G, et al. A randomised pilot study to assess the efficacy of an interactive, multimedial tool of cognitive stimulation in Alzheimer's disease. *Neurol Neurosurg Psychiatry.* 2006;77:1116–1121.
13. Ramakrishnan S, Pollack ME. Intelligent monitoring in a robotic assistant for the elderly. *Proceedings of the 16th National Conference on Artificial Intelligence,* Orlando, FL, 2000.
14. Gould, D. Video: Robots help dementia patients. *Griffith University News.* Retrieved January 2013 from http://app.griffith.edu.au/news/2013/01/03/video-robots-help-dementia-patients/.
15. Mordoch E, Osterreicher A, Guse L, Roger K, Thompson G. Use of social commitment robots in the care of elderly people with dementia: a literature review. *Maturitas.* 2013;74:14–20.
16. Wada K, Shibata T, Musha T, Kimura S. Effects of robot therapy for demented patients evaluated EEG. *Proc IEEE/RSJ Int Conf IROS.* 2005:2205–2210.
17. Broekens J, Heerink M, Rosendal H. Assistive social robots in elderly care: a review. *Gerontechnology.* 2009;8:94–103.
18. Libin AV, Libin EV. Person-robot interactions from the robopsychologists' point of view: the robotic psychology and robotherapy approach. *Proc IEEE.* 2004;92:1789–1803.
19. Topo P. Technology study to meet the needs of people with dementia and their caregivers: a literature review. *J Appl Gerontol.* 2012;28:5–37.
20. Bemelmans R, Gelderblom J, Jonker P, de Witt L. Social assistive robots in elderly care: a systematic review into effects and effectiveness. *Am Med Dir Assoc.* 2012;13:114–120.
21. Alm N, Astell A, Ellis M, Dye R, Gowans G, Campbell JA. Cognitive prosthesis and communication support for people with dementia. *Neuropsych Rehab.* 2004;14:117–134.
22. Zanetti O, Zanieri G, Vreese LPD, Frisoni G, Binetti G. *Utilizing an Electronic Memory Aid With Alzheimer's Disease Patients. A Study of Feasibility.* Presentation at the Sixth International Stockholm/Springfield Symposium on Advances in Alzheimer Therapy. Stockholm, Sweden, 2000.

23. Mihailidis A, Fernie G, Barbenel JC. The use of artificial intelligence in the design of an intelligent cognitive orthotic for people with dementia. *Assist Tech*. 2001;13:23–39.
24. Hodges S, Williams L, Berry E, et al. SenseCam: a retrospective memory aid. In: Dourish P, Friday A, eds, *Ubicomp, LNCS 4206*. 2006:177–193.
25. McKeown J, Clarke A, Ingleton C, Ryan T, Repper J. The use of life story work with people with dementia to enhance person-centered care. *Int J Older People Nurs*. 2010;5:148–158.
26. Thompson R. Using life story work to enhance care. *Nursing Older People*. 2011;23:16–21.
27. Mynatt ED, Essa I, Rogers W. *Increasing Opportunities for Aging in Place*. ACM Conference on Universal Usability, Washington, DC. New York: ACM Press; 2000:65–71.
28. Gilley DW, Wilson RS, Bennett DA, et al. Cessation of driving and unsafe motor vehicle operation by dementia patients. *Arch Intern Med*. 1991;151:941–946.
29. Bright R. The use of music therapy and activities with dementia patients who are deemed "difficult to manage." *Clin Gerontol*. 1986;6:131–144.
30. Summer L. Guided imagery and music with the elderly. *Mus Ther*. 1981;1:39–42.
31. Christie ME. Music therapy applications in a skilled and intermediate care nursing home.
32. Helmes E, Wiancko D. *Effects of Music in Reducing Disruptive Behavior in a General Hospital*. Paper presented at the 16th Congress of the International Association of Gerontology, Adelaide, Australia, 1997.
33. Gerdner L, Swanson E. Effects of individualized music on confused and agitated elderly patients. *Arch Psychiatric Nurs*. 1993;7:284–291.
34. Thomas WH. *Life Worth Living*. Acton, MA: VanderWyk & Burnham; 1996.
35. Resnick O, Ransom S. The search for Eden: an alternative path for nursing homes. *Long-Term Care Interface*. 2001;2:45–48.
36. Bergman-Evans B. Beyond the basics: effects of the Eden Alternative model on quality of life issues. *J Gerontol Nurs*. 2004;30:27–34.
37. Van Ort S, Phillips L. Feeding nursing home residents with Alzheimer's disease. *Geriatr Nurs*. 1992;13:249–253.

38. Sloane PD, Davidson S, Buckwalter K, et al. Management of the patient with disruptive vocalization. *Gerontologist.* 1997;37: 675–682.
39. Smith M, Filips J. Info-Connect. Disruptive vocalizations. Iowa Geriatric Education Center: The University of Iowa; 2009. Retrieved April 10, 2013 from http://www.healthcare.uiowa .edu/igec/publications/info-connect/assets/disruptive _vocalizations.pdf.

Index